CERTIFIED MEDICAL ASSISTANT

EXAM PREP

By

John Bill, PharmD

Table of Contents   Pages

PART ONE

Questions...4

Answers to part 1...31

PART TWO

Questions...43

Answers to part 2...69

PART THREE

Questions...81

Answers to part 3...102

PART FOUR

Questions...114

Answers to part 4 139

PART FIVE

Questions...150

Answers to part 5 177

PART SIX

Questions...187

Answers to part 6 212

PART SEVEN

Questions...224

Answers to part 7 258

PART EIGHT

Questions...270

Answers to part 8...296

PART NINE

Questions...311

Answers to part 9 345

PART TEN

Questions...361

Answers to part 10 386

PART ELEVEN

Questions...400

Answers to part 11...426

PART TWELVE

Questions...435

Answers to part 12 460

MEDICAL ASSISTANT CERTIFICATION
EXAMINATION STUDY GUIDE
PART-ONE

1. What is the definition of ethics?

    a. Rules of conduct made by a government body.

    b. Knowledge of what is right conduct versus what is wrong conduct.

    c. Concerned with offenses against the public.

    d. All

2. What should you do if you suspect a patient is being abused?

    a. Ignore the situation and continue providing care as usual.

    b. Report the situation to the patient's family.

    c. Share/report concerns to the RN immediately.

    d. None

3. What is the difference between criminal laws and civil laws?

    a. Criminal laws are concerned with relationships between people, while civil laws are concerned with offenses against the public.

    b. Criminal laws are concerned with offenses against the public, while civil laws are concerned with relationships between people.

    c. Criminal laws and civil laws are the same thing.

    d. A and B are answer

4. What are the principles that guide ethics in the medical field?

    a. Discrimination, responsibility, and self-discipline.

    b. Integrity, responsibility to service and community, respect, self-discipline, and intent to

        further your career.

    c. Responsibility, respect, and intent to further your career.

    d. All

5. What is the Patient Care Partnership?

    a. A guide for physicians involved in patient care.

    b. A guide for patients and physicians involved in patient care.

    c. A document outlining a patient's medical history.

    d. All answer except a

6. What is a patient's right regarding treatment without discrimination?

    a. To receive treatment only if they can pay for it.

    b. To receive treatment without discrimination as to race, color, religion, gender, national

        origin, disability, or source of payment.

    c. To receive treatment only if they are of a certain religion.

    d. None

7. What information should a patient receive before giving informed consent for a procedure or treatment?

    a. No information is necessary.

    b. Only the benefits of the procedure or treatment.

    c. All the information they need, including the possible risks and benefits of the procedure or treatment.

    d. All

8. What is a patient's right regarding refusing treatment, examination, or observation?

    a. They have no right to refuse.

    b. They have the right to refuse but will be forced to undergo the procedure or treatment anyway.

    c. They have the right to refuse and be told what effect this may have on their health.

    d. None

9. Which government program provides insurance for persons over 65?

    a. Medicaid

    b. TRICARE

    c. Medicare

    d. CHAMPVA

10. What does it mean to self-insure?

    a. To have no insurance coverage.

    b. To purchase insurance from a private company.

    c. For employers to pay directly for employees' medical bills.

    d. To receive insurance coverage from the government.

11. What is the purpose of Medicare Part B?

    a. To pay for inpatient hospital care.

    b. To provide voluntary Medicare prescription drug plans.

    c. To offer Medicare Advantage plans that compete with the Original Medicare Plan.

    d. To help pay for physician services.

12. What is TRICARE?

    a. Insurance for low-income people.

    b. Insurance for active duty and retired service personnel and their families.

    c. Insurance for veterans with service-related disabilities.

    d. A program that pays for inpatient hospital care.

13. What is co-insurance?

   a. A fixed amount that a patient pays for a medical service.

   b. A percentage of the charge that a patient pays for a medical service.

   c. A payment made by an insurance company to a healthcare provider.

   d. A program that provides coverage for employees for job-related illnesses or injuries.

14. What are standard precautions used for?

   a. To prevent transmission of diseases through the air

   b. To prevent transmission of diseases through food

   c. To prevent transmission of diseases through contact with blood, body fluids, non-intact skin, and mucous membranes

   d. To prevent transmission of diseases through physical contact

15. When should standard precautions be used?

   a. Only when a patient is known to be infectious.

   b. Only when a patient is showing symptoms of an infection.

   c. When providing care to all individuals, whether or not they appear infectious or symptomatic.

   d. Only when providing care to individuals with compromised immune systems

16. What is the most important procedure for preventing cross-contamination?

   a. Wearing gloves

   b. Wearing a mask

   c. Washing hands

   d. Using hand sanitizer

17. When should gloves be worn?

   a. Only when performing invasive procedures

   b. Only when touching broken skin or mucous membranes

   c. Only when handling contaminated waste materials

   d. Before touching anything wet, including broken skin, mucous membranes, blood or other body fluids, or soiled instruments and contaminated waste materials

18. What should be considered when providing care to individuals?

   a. Only their visible symptoms

   b. Only their medical history

   c. Only their age and gender

   d. Every person (patient or staff) as potentially infectious and susceptible to infection

19. What are airborne precautions designed to reduce the transmission of?

    a.   Pathogens spread wholly or partly by droplets larger than 0.001 mm in size.

    b.   Particles 0.001mm or less in size can remain in the air for several hours and be widely dispersed.

    c.   Pathogens that can be acquired by contact with blood, body fluids, non-intact skin, and mucous membranes.

    d.   Pathogens that can be acquired through physical contact.

20. What is required to prevent airborne transmission?

    a.   Special air handling and ventilation

    b.   Wearing a mask

    c.   Scrubbing instruments with special brushes and detergent

    d.   Disinfecting surfaces with a cleaning solution

21. What are droplet precautions designed to reduce the transmission of?

    a.   Pathogens that can be acquired by contact with blood, body fluids, non-intact skin, and mucous membranes.

    b.   Particles 0.001mm or less in size can remain in the air for several hours and be widely dispersed.

    c.   Pathogens spread wholly or partly by droplets larger than 0.001 mm in size.

    d.   Pathogens that can be acquired through physical contact.

22. What is recommended to reduce the incidence of infection when interacting with patients?

    a. Scrubbing instruments with special brushes and detergent

    b. Disinfecting surfaces with a cleaning solution

    c. Wearing gloves

    d. Wearing a mask

23. What is the process of destroying all microbial forms of life?

    a. Sanitization

    b. Disinfection

    c. Sterilization

    d. Autoclaving

24. What is asepsis?

    a. The process of becoming unclean

    b. The practice of removing or destroying pathogens

    c. The process of destroying all microbes

    d. The process of transmitting pathogens

25. What is surgical asepsis?

    a. The practice of removing or destroying pathogens

    b. The practice of keeping items free of all microbes

    c. The process of becoming unclean

    d. The process of destroying pathogens

26. What is sterilization?

    a. The process of becoming unclean

    b. The process of destroying pathogens

    c. The practice of removing or destroying pathogens

    d. The practice of keeping items free of all microbes

27. What is the most common way of transmitting pathogens?

    a. Through the air

    b. Through contaminated food and water

    c. By touching a contaminated item

    d. Through physical contact with an infected person

28. What are vital signs?

    a. The process of becoming unclean

    b. The heartbeat, breathing rate, temperature, and blood pressure.

    c. The practice of removing or destroying pathogens

    d. The practice of keeping items free of all microbes

29. Which agency regulates controlled substances in the United States?

    a. FDA

    b. DEA

    c. CDC

    d. NIH

30. Which category of drugs relieves mild to severe pain?

    a.   Analgesics

    b.   Anesthetics

    c.   Antibiotics

    d.   Anticoagulants

31. Which category of drugs prevents sensation of pain?

    a.   Analgesics

    b.   Anesthetics

    c.   Antibiotics

    d.   Anticoagulants

32. Which category of drugs kills bacterial microorganisms?

    a.   Analgesics

    b.   Anesthetics

    c.   Antibiotics

    d.   Anticoagulants

33. Which category of drugs prevents blood from clotting?

    a.   Analgesics

    b.   Anesthetics

    c.   Antibiotics

    d.   Anticoagulants

34. Which category of drugs reduces blood pressure and increases urine output?

    a.   Analgesics

    b.   Anesthetics

    c.   Antibiotics

    d.   Diuretics

35. Which category of drugs constricts blood vessels and increases blood pressure?

    a.   Analgesics

    b.   Anesthetics

    c.   Antibiotics

    d.   Vasoconstrictors

36. What is the term for two drugs working together?

    a.   Synergist

    b.   Antagonist

    c.   Adverse reaction

    d.   Dosage

37. What is the term for one drug decreasing the effect of another?

    a.   Synergist

    b.   Antagonist

    c.   Adverse reaction

    d.   Dosage

38. What is the most commonly used system of measurement for pharmacology and drug administration in the United States?

    a.   Metric system

    b.   Apothecary system

    c.   Household system

    d.   Imperial system

39. What is the layer or sac that surrounds the heart called?

    a.   Myocardium

    b.   Endocardium

    c.   Epicardium

    d.   Pericardium

40. What is the middle layer of the heart called?

    a.   Myocardium

    b.   Endocardium

    c.   Epicardium

    d.   Pericardium

41. What is the innermost layer of the heart called?

    a.   Myocardium

    b.   Endocardium

    c.   Epicardium

    d.   Pericardium

42. What is the top layer of the heart called?

    a.   Myocardium

    b.   Endocardium

    c.   Epicardium

    d.   Pericardium

43. What is the system responsible for the regulation of the pumping action of the heart?

    a.   Respiratory system

    b.   Digestive system

    c.   Nervous system

    d.   Conduction system

44. What causes the myocardium to contract?

    a.   Electrical impulses

    b.   Chemical signals

    c.   Hormones

    d.   Mechanical pressure

45. What is the term for the rate and rhythm of the heart?

    a.   Excitability

    b.   Conductivity

    c.   Contractility

    d.   Cardiac cycle

46. What is the term for the cells responsible for regulating the heart rate and rhythm?

    a. Pacemaker cells

    b. Muscle cells

    c. Nerve cells

    d. Epithelial cells

47. What is the term for the pathway that the electrical impulse travels through in the heart?

    a. Intermodal pathway

    b. Interventricular pathway

    c. Interatrial pathway

    d. Intraventricular pathway

48. Where does the conduction system of the heart begin?

    a. Atrioventricular (AV) node

    b. Purkinje fibers

    c. Sinoatrial (SA) node

    d. Bundle of His

49. What is cardiac output?

    a. The amount of blood pumped by the heart per minute.

    b. A condition caused by a lack of oxygen-rich blood in the heart.

    c. An abnormal sound that may indicate valvular heart disease.

    d. A tool used to record the electrical activity of the heart.

50. What is myocardial infarction?

    a. A condition caused by a lack of oxygen-rich blood in the heart.

    b. An obstruction to the myocardial tissue that causes heart cells to die.

    c. An abnormal sound that may indicate valvular heart disease.

    d. A tool used to record the electrical activity of the heart.

51. What is myocardial ischemia?

    a. The amount of blood pumped by the heart per minute.

    b. A condition caused by a lack of oxygen-rich blood in the heart.

    c. An obstruction to the myocardial tissue that causes heart cells to die.

    d. An abnormal sound that may indicate valvular heart disease.

52. What is a murmur?

    a. The amount of blood pumped by the heart per minute.

    b. A condition caused by a lack of oxygen-rich blood in the heart.

    c. An abnormal sound that may indicate valvular heart disease.

    d. A tool used to record.

53. What is arrhythmia?

    a. The amount of blood pumped by the heart per minute.

    b. A condition caused by a lack of oxygen-rich blood in the heart.

    c. An abnormal sound that may indicate valvular heart disease.

    d. Any disorder of your heart rate or rhythm

54. What is an electrocardiogram?

    a.   The amount of blood pumped by the heart per minute.

    b.   A condition caused by a lack of oxygen-rich blood in the heart.

    c.   A tool used to record the electrical activity of the heart.

    d.   An abnormal sound that may indicate valvular heart disease.

55. What is an electrocardiograph?

    a.   A device that amplifies low-voltage electric impulses detected on the skin and produces a printed record of that electrical activity.

    b.   A condition caused by a lack of oxygen-rich blood in the heart.

    c.   An abnormal sound that may indicate valvular heart disease.

    d.   A tool used to record the electrical activity of the heart.

56. What is necessary to perform an electrocardiogram?

    a.   Placing electrodes on the patient's skin

    b.   Administering medication to the patient

    c.   Performing surgery on the patient

    d.   None of the above

57. What are electrodes?

    a.   Adhesive pads containing conductive gel.

    b.   A device that amplifies low-voltage electric impulses detected on the skin and produces a printed record of that electrical activity.

    c.   Color-coded wires that connect to the electrocardiograph

    d.   An abnormal sound that may indicate valvular heart disease.

58. What is a cardiac monitor?

   a. A device that amplifies low-voltage electric impulses detected on the skin and produces a printed record of that electrical activity.

   b. A tool used to record the electrical activity of the heart.

   c. An abnormal sound that may indicate valvular heart disease.

   d. The amount of blood pumped by the heart per minute.

59. What is asystole?

   a. Organized electrical activity that should result in a pulse but there is no pulse.

   b. Any electric activity on an EGC that is non-cardiac in origin.

   c. Total absence of cardiac activity (Flat line)

   d. The liquid portion of the blood that remains after the blood has coagulated.

60. What is pulseless electrical activity?

   a. Organized electrical activity that should result in a pulse but there is no pulse.

   b. Any electric activity on an EGC that is non-cardiac in origin.

   c. Total absence of cardiac activity (Flat line)

   d. The liquid portion of the blood that remains after the blood has coagulated.

61. What are artifacts?

   a. Organized electrical activity that should result in a pulse but there is no pulse.

   b. Any electric activity on an EGC that is non-cardiac in origin.

   c. Total absence of cardiac activity (Flat line)

   d. The liquid portion of the blood that remains after the blood has coagulated.

62. What is the purpose of The National Committee for Clinical Laboratory Standards (NCCLS)?

    a.   To set standards for phlebotomy programs

    b.   To regulate the amount of blood within the body of the average human adult

    c.   To produce hemoglobin, the pigment responsible for the reddish color of the blood

    d.   To categorize white blood cells into five different types

63. How much blood is within the body of the average human adult?

    a.   1-2 liters

    b.   3-4 liters

    c.   5-6 liters

    d.   7-8 liters

64. What is serum?

    a.   The liquid portion of the blood in its anticoagulated state

    b.   The liquid portion of the blood that remains after the blood has coagulated.

    c.   The pigment responsible for the reddish color of the blood

    d.   The category of white blood cells that fights infections.

65. What are red blood cells?

    a.   The liquid portion of the blood in its anticoagulated state

    b.   The liquid portion of the blood that remains after the blood has coagulated.

    c.   The category of white blood cells that fights infections.

    d.   The cells that contain hemoglobin and are responsible for the reddish color of the blood.

66. What are white blood cells?

    a.   The liquid portion of the blood in its anticoagulated state

    b.   The liquid portion of the blood that remains after the blood has coagulated.

    c.   The cells that contain hemoglobin and are responsible for the reddish color of the blood.

    d.   The category of blood cells that fight infections is categorized into five different types.

67. How long do red blood cells live?

    a.   Approximately 30 days

    b.   Approximately 60 days

    c.   Approximately 90 days

    d.   Approximately 120 days

68. What is hemoglobin?

    a.   The liquid portion of the blood in its anticoagulated state

    b.   The liquid portion of the blood that remains after the blood has coagulated.

    c.   The pigment responsible for the reddish color of the blood

    d.   The category of white blood cells that fights infections.

69. What is a random urine specimen used for?

    a.   Testing for pH

    b.   Testing for glucose or ketones

    c.   Testing for blood

    d.   Urinalysis

70. What is a midstream specimen?

    a. A specimen collected anytime for urinalysis.

    b. A specimen collected during a 24-hour period.

    c. A specimen collected after cleaning the perineal area.

    d. A specimen collected after fasting for 12 hours.

71. What is a 24-hour specimen?

    a. A specimen collected anytime for urinalysis.

    b. A specimen collected during a 24-hour period.

    c. A specimen collected after cleaning the perineal area.

    d. A specimen collected after fasting for 12 hours.

72. What is the purpose of testing for pH in urine?

    a. To measure if urine is acidic or alkaline.

    b. To test for glucose or ketones

    c. To test for blood

    d. To perform a routine urinalysis

73. What is glycosuria?

    a. The appearance of sugar in the urine

    b. The appearance of acetone in the urine

    c. The appearance of blood in the urine

    d. The appearance of protein in the urine

74. What is a double-voided specimen?

    a. A specimen collected anytime for urinalysis.

    b. A specimen collected during a 24-hour period.

    c. A specimen collected after cleaning the perineal area.

    d. A specimen collected after voiding, waiting a few minutes, and then voiding again.

75. What is hematuria?

    a. The appearance of sugar in the urine

    b. The appearance of acetone in the urine

    c. The appearance of blood in the urine

    d. The appearance of protein in the urine

76. What can cause blood to appear in the urine?

    a. Injuries or illnesses

    b. Fasting for 12 hours

    c. Drinking too much water

    d. Taking certain medications

77. What can cause blood to appear in stools?

    a. Ulcers, some forms of cancer, or hemorrhoids

    b. Drinking too much water

    c. Taking certain medications

    d. Fasting for 12 hours

78. What should be followed when testing stool?

    a. The doctor's prescription request

    b. The patient's preference

    c. The time of day

    d. The type of food consumed.

79. Which tube is commonly used for serum determinations in chemistry testing and blood bank testing?

    a. Blue

    b. Lavender

    c. Green

    d. Red

80. Which additive is used in the blue tube to prevent coagulation by binding calcium?

    a. EDTA

    b. Heparin

    c. Sodium citrate

    d. Sodium fluoride

81. Why is it advised to draw 2 to 3 ml of blood in a tube without additives before drawing the blue tube?

    a. To prevent contamination

    b. To ensure enough blood is collected.

    c. To prevent coagulation

    d. To ensure accurate test results

82. Which tube is commonly used for coagulation tests and heparin therapy?

   a. Blue

   b. Lavender

   c. Green

   d. Red

83. Which additive is used in the lavender tube to bind the calcium needed for clot formation?

   a. EDTA

   b. Heparin

   c. Sodium citrate

   d. Sodium fluoride

84. Which tube is commonly used for hematology testing and ESR testing?

   a. Blue

   b. Lavender

   c. Green

   d. Red

85. Which additive is used in the green tube as a natural anticoagulant that inhibits thrombin?

   a. EDTA

   b. Heparin

   c. Sodium citrate

   d. Sodium fluoride

86. Which tube is commonly used for routine chemistry testing?

    a. Blue

    b. Lavender

    c. Green

    d. Red

87. Which additives are used in the gray tube for glucose tolerance and lactic acid measurement?

    a. Sodium citrate and EDTA

    b. Heparin and sodium citrate

    c. Sodium fluoride and potassium oxalate

    d. EDTA and heparin

88. Which tube is commonly used for glucose tolerance and lactic acid measurement?

    a. Blue

    b. Lavender

    c. Green

    d. Gray

89. Which department in the medical laboratory deals with the handling of various blood specimens?

    a. Hematology Section

    b. Chemistry Section

    c. Blood Bank Section

    d. Anatomical Pathology Section

90. Which tests are commonly performed in the Hematology Section?

    a. Blood glucose levels

    b. Electrolytes (sodium, potassium, chloride)

    c. WBC counts, RBC counts, hemoglobin, hematocrit (Hct), RBC indices, and platelet counts

    d. None of the above

91. What do the results of tests performed in the Hematology Section indicate?

    a. Pregnancy confirmation

    b. Liver disorder

    c. Dehydration, anemia, leukemia, and a wide variety of other diseases

    d. None of the above

92. Which department in the medical laboratory performs tests for blood glucose levels and electrolytes?

    a. Hematology Section

    b. Chemistry Section

    c. Blood Bank Section

    d. Anatomical Pathology Section

93. What can the results of tests performed in the Chemistry Section indicate?

    a. Dehydration, anemia, leukemia, and a wide variety of other diseases

    b. Pregnancy confirmation

    c. Presence of a liver disorder

    d. None of the above

94. Which section of the laboratory collects, stores, and prepares blood for transfusion?

    a. Hematology Section

    b. Chemistry Section

    c. Blood Bank Section

    d. Anatomical Pathology Section

95. What is essential for all staff members to comply with in the Blood Bank Section?

    a. Standards for patient identification and specimen handling

    b. Standards for surgical and anatomical pathology analysis

    c. Standards for diagnostic testing

    d. None of the above

96. Which of the following is not a test commonly performed in the Hematology Section?

    a. WBC counts

    b. RBC counts

    c. Electrolytes (sodium, potassium, chloride)

    d. Platelet counts.

97. What do the results of tests performed in the Blood Bank Section indicate?

    a. Dehydration, anemia, leukemia, and a wide variety of other diseases

    b. Pregnancy confirmation

    c. Blood type and compatibility for transfusion

    d. None of the above

98. Which section of the laboratory deals with surgical and anatomical pathology analysis?

   a.   Hematology Section

   b.   Chemistry Section

   c.   Blood Bank Section

   d.   Anatomical Pathology Section

99. Which tests are commonly performed in the Chemistry Section?

   a.   WBC counts, RBC counts, hemoglobin, hematocrit (Hct), RBC indices, and platelet

        counts

   b.   Blood type and compatibility for transfusion

   c.   Blood glucose levels, electrolytes (sodium, potassium, chloride), total protein, etc.

   d.   None of the above

100. What is the purpose of the Hematology Section in the medical laboratory?

   a.   To collect, store, and prepare blood for transfusion.

   b.   To perform surgical and anatomical pathology analysis

   c.   To handle various blood specimens and perform tests for conditions such as dehydration,

        anemia, leukemia, and a wide variety of other diseases.

   d.   None of the above

PART- ONE

ANSWER TO MEDICAL ASSISTANT QUESTIONS

1. **Answer: B**

    - Knowledge of what is right conduct versus what is wrong conduct.

2. **Answer: C**

    - Share/report concerns to the RN immediately. This is because it is the ethical duty of a healthcare worker to report any suspected abuse to the appropriate authorities.

3. **Answer: B**

    - Criminal laws are concerned with offenses against the public, while civil laws are concerned with relationships between people. This means that criminal laws deal with crimes that are considered harmful to society as a whole, while civil laws deal with disputes between individuals or organizations.

4. **Answer: B**

    - Integrity, responsibility to service and community, respect, self-discipline, and intent to further your career: These are the principles that guide ethics in the medical field. They include being honest and trustworthy, serving the community, showing respect for patients and colleagues, being self-disciplined, and having a commitment to furthering your career.

5. **Answer B**

    - A guide for patients and physicians involved in patient care: The Patient Care Partnership is a guide that outlines the rights and responsibilities of patients and physicians involved in patient care.

6. **Answer B**

    - To receive treatment without discrimination as to race, color, religion, gender, national origin, disability, or source of payment: This is a patient's right to receive treatment without being discriminated against based on their race, color, religion, gender, national origin, disability, or ability to pay.

7. **Answer C**

    - All the information they need, including the possible risks and benefits of the procedure or treatment: Before giving informed consent for a procedure or treatment, a patient should receive all the information they need, including the possible risks and benefits of the procedure or treatment.

8. **Answer C**

- They have the right to refuse and be told what effect this may have on their health: A patient has the right to refuse treatment, examination, or observation, and they should be informed of the potential consequences of their decision on their health.

9. **Answer C**

- Medicare

- A government program that provides insurance for persons over 65.

10. **Answer C**

- Self-insure -

- For employers to pay directly for employees' medical bills.

11. **Answer D**

- **Medicare Part B**

- Supplementary Medical Insurance that helps pay for physician services.

12. **Answer B**

- **TRICARE**

- Insurance for active duty and retired service personnel and their families.

13. **Answer B**

- **Co-insurance**

- A percentage of the charge that a patient pays for a medical service.

14. **Answer C**

- **Standard precautions**

- A set of infection control practices used to prevent transmission of diseases that can be acquired by contact with blood, body fluids, non-intact skin, and mucous membranes.

15. **Answer C**

- **When to use standard precautions**

- When providing care to all individuals, whether or not they appear infectious or symptomatic.

16. **Answer C**

- Most important procedure for preventing cross-contamination - Washing hands.

17. **Answer D**

- **When to wear gloves**

- Before touching anything wet, including broken skin, mucous membranes, blood or other body fluids, or soiled instruments and contaminated waste materials.

18. **Answer D**

- What to consider when providing care to individuals - Every person (patient or staff) as potentially infectious and susceptible to infection.

19. **Answer B**

- **Airborne precautions**

- Precautions designed to reduce the transmission of particles 0.001mm or less in size that can remain in the air for several hours and be widely dispersed. Special air handling and ventilation are required to prevent airborne transmission.

20. **Answer A**

- **Special air handling and ventilation**

- A system of air circulation and filtration that is designed to prevent the spread of airborne pathogens by removing contaminated air and replacing it with clean air.

21. **Answer C**

- **Droplet precautions.**

- Precautions designed to reduce the transmission of pathogens spread wholly or partly by droplets larger than 0.001 mm in size. Pathogens are microbes that can cause disease.

22. **Answer D**

- **Wearing a mask**

- A protective measure that can reduce the incidence of infection when interacting with patients by preventing the spread of droplets from the mouth and nose.

23. Answer C

- **Sterilization**

- The process of destroying all microbial forms of life. This is typically achieved using an autoclave, which uses high pressure and high temperature steam to kill all microorganisms.

24. Answer B

- The practice of removing or destroying pathogens - Asepsis is the practice of removing or destroying disease-causing microorganisms, such as bacteria, viruses, and fungi, to prevent the spread of infection.

25. Answer B

- The practice of keeping items free of all microbes - Surgical asepsis is the practice of keeping surgical instruments, equipment, and the surgical environment free of all microorganisms to prevent surgical site infections.

26. Answer B

- The process of destroying pathogens - Sterilization is the process of destroying all microorganisms, including bacteria, viruses, and fungi, to prevent the spread of infection.

27. Answer C

- By touching a contaminated item - Pathogens can be transmitted through contact with contaminated surfaces, objects, or equipment, making it important to practice good hand hygiene and disinfection protocols.

28. Answer B

- The heartbeat, breathing rate, temperature, and blood pressure - Vital signs are measurements of the body's basic functions, including heart rate, respiratory rate, body temperature, and blood pressure, which can provide important information about a person's overall health and well-being.

29.Answer B

- Agency regulates controlled substances in the United States- The Drug Enforcement Administration (DEA) is the agency responsible for regulating controlled substances in the United States.

30. Answer A

- category of drugs relieves mild to severe pain- Analgesics are a category of drugs that relieve mild to severe pain, such as Tylenol and aspirin.

31. Answer B

- category of drugs prevents sensation of pain - Anesthetics are a category of drugs that prevent the sensation of pain, such as lidocaine.

32. Answer C

- category of drugs kills bacterial microorganisms - Antibiotics are a category of drugs that kill bacterial microorganisms, such as amoxicillin, ciprofloxacin, and azithromycin.

33. Answer D

- category of drugs prevents blood from clotting - Anticoagulants are a category of drugs that prevent blood from clotting, such as Lovenox, heparin sodium, and warfarin sodium.

34. Answer D

- Category of drugs reduces blood pressure and increases urine output - Diuretics are a category of drugs that reduce blood pressure and increase urine output, and there are various names for them.

35. Answer D

- category of drugs constricts blood vessels and increases blood pressure - Vasoconstrictors are a category of drugs that constrict blood vessels and increase blood pressure.

36. Answer A

- The term for two drugs working together - Synergist is the term for two drugs working together to produce a greater effect than either drug alone.

37. Answer B

- The term for one drug decreasing the effect of another - Antagonist is the term for one drug decreasing the effect of another drug.

38. Answer A

- **The most commonly used system of measurement for pharmacology and drug administration in** the United States - The metric system is the most commonly used system of measurement for pharmacology and drug administration in the United States, using liters to measure volumes and grams to measure weight.

39. Answer D

- The layer or sac that surrounds the heart is called - The pericardium is a double-layered sac that surrounds the heart and protects it from infection and trauma.

40. Answer A

- The middle layer of the heart is called - The myocardium is the muscular middle layer of the heart that contracts and pumps blood throughout the body.

41. Answer B

- The innermost layer of the heart is called - The endocardium is the thin, smooth innermost layer of the heart that lines the chambers and valves.

42. Answer C

- The top layer of the heart is called - The epicardium is the outermost layer of the heart that covers the surface of the heart and is also known as the visceral layer of the pericardium.

43. Answer D

- The system responsible for the regulation of the pumping action of the heart - The conduction system is a group of specialized cells that generate and transmit electrical impulses to regulate the heartbeat.

44. Answer A

- causes the myocardium to contract - Electrical impulses generated by the conduction system cause the myocardium to contract and pump blood.

45. Answer D

- The term for the rate and rhythm of the heart - The cardiac cycle is the term for the sequence of events that occur during one heartbeat, including the contraction and relaxation of the heart chambers.

46. Answer A

- The term for the cells responsible for regulating the heart rate and rhythm - Pacemaker cells are specialized cells in the sinoatrial (SA) node that generate electrical impulses to regulate the heart rate and rhythm.

47. Answer A

- The term for the pathway that the electrical impulse travels through in the heart - The conduction pathway is a network of specialized cells that transmit electrical impulses through the heart, including the SA node, AV node, bundle of His, and Purkinje fibers.

48. Answer C

- Where does the conduction system of the heart begin? - The conduction system of the heart begins in the sinoatrial (SA) node, which is located in the right atrium and generates electrical impulses to regulate the heartbeat.

49. Answer A

- **Cardiac output**

- Cardiac output is the amount of blood pumped by the heart per minute.

50. Answer B

- **Myocardial infarction**

- Myocardial infarction, commonly known as a heart attack, is a term that refers to an obstruction to the myocardial tissue. This obstruction causes an interruption of the blood supply to part of the heart which causes the heart cells to die.

51. Answer B

- **Myocardial ischemia**

- Myocardial ischemia, also known as angina, is a condition caused by a lack of oxygen-rich blood in the heart.

52. Answer C

- **murmur**

- A murmur is an abnormal sound that may indicate valvular heart disease.

53. Answer D

- **Arrhythmia - Arrhythmia is a term used to refer to any disorder of your heart rate or rhythm.**

54. Answer C

- An electrocardiogram - An electrocardiogram, also known as the ECG or EKG, is a tool used to record the electrical activity of the heart.

55. Answer A

- An electrocardiograph - An electrocardiograph is a device that amplifies low-voltage electric impulses detected on the skin and produces a printed record of that electrical activity.

56. Answer A

- Necessary perform an electrocardiogram - In order to perform an electrocardiogram, it is necessary to place electrodes, adhesive pads containing a conductive gel, on the patient's skin.

57. Answer A

- **Electrodes**

- Electrodes are adhesive pads containing a conductive gel that are placed on the patient's skin to record the electrical activity of the heart.

58. Answer A

- A cardiac monitor

- A cardiac monitor is a device that amplifies low-voltage electric impulses detected on the skin and produces a printed record of that electrical activity.

59. Answer: C

- **Total absence of cardiac activity (Flat line)**

60. Answer: A

- Organized electrical activity that should result in a pulse but there is no pulse.

61. Answer: B

- **Any electric activity on an EGC that is non-cardiac in origin.**

62. Answer: A

- **To set standards for phlebotomy programs**

63. Answer: C

- **5-6 liters**

64. Answer: B

- The liquid portion of the blood that remains after the blood has coagulated.

65. Answer: D

- The cells that contain hemoglobin and are responsible for the reddish color of the blood.

66. Answer: D

- The category of blood cells that fight infections is categorized into five different types.

67. Answer: D

- Approximately 120 days

68. Answer: C

- The pigment responsible for the reddish color of the blood

69. Answer D

- Urinalysis - A laboratory test that examines the physical, chemical, and microscopic properties of urine to diagnose and monitor various medical conditions.

70. Answer C

- A specimen collected after cleaning the perineal area - A midstream specimen, also known as a clean-voided specimen or a clean-catch specimen, is a urine sample collected after cleaning the perineal area to avoid contamination.

71. Answer B

- A specimen collected during a 24-hour period - A 24-hour urine collection is a laboratory test that measures the number of certain substances in urine over a 24-hour period.

72. Answer A

- To measure if urine is acidic or alkaline - Testing for pH in urine is a laboratory test that measures the acidity or alkalinity of urine.

73. Answer A

- The appearance of sugar in the urine - Glycosuria is a medical condition characterized by the presence of glucose (sugar) in the urine.

74. Answer D

- A specimen collected after voiding, waiting a few minutes, and then voiding again - A double-voided specimen is a urine sample collected after voiding, waiting a few minutes, and then voiding again to obtain a more accurate measurement of certain substances in urine.

75. Answer C

- The appearance of blood in the urine - Hematuria is a medical condition characterized by the presence of blood in the urine.

76. Answer A

- Injuries or illnesses - Blood in the urine can be caused by various medical conditions, such as infections, kidney stones, tumors, or trauma.

77. Answer A

- Ulcers, some forms of cancer, or hemorrhoids - Blood in the stool can be caused by various medical conditions, such as ulcers, colon cancer, hemorrhoids, or inflammatory bowel disease.

78. Answer. A

- The doctor's prescription request - When testing stool, it is important to follow the doctor's prescription request to obtain accurate results and diagnose medical conditions.

79. Answer. D

- Red: The red tube is used for serum determinations in chemistry testing and blood bank testing. It does not contain any additives.

80. Answer C

- Sodium citrate: The blue tube contains sodium citrate as an additive, which prevents coagulation by binding calcium.

81. Answer C

- To prevent coagulation: It is advised to draw 2 to 3 ml of blood in a tube without additives before drawing the blue tube to prevent coagulation.

82. Answer A

- Blue: The blue tube is commonly used for coagulation tests and heparin therapy. It contains sodium citrate as an additive.

83. Answer A

- EDTA: The lavender tube contains EDTA as an additive, which binds the calcium needed for clot formation.

84. Answer B

- Lavender: The lavender tube is commonly used for hematology testing and ESR testing. It contains EDTA as an additive.

85. Answer B

- Heparin: The green tube contains heparin as an additive, which is a natural anticoagulant that inhibits thrombin.

86. Answer C

- Green: The green tube is commonly used for routine chemistry testing. It contains heparin as an additive.

87. Answer C

- Sodium fluoride and potassium oxalate: The gray tube contains sodium fluoride as a preservative that inhibits glycolytic action and potassium oxalate as an anticoagulant that binds calcium. It is commonly used for glucose tolerance and lactic acid measurement.

88. Answer D

- Gray: The gray tube is commonly used for glucose tolerance and lactic acid measurement. It contains sodium fluoride and potassium oxalate as additives.

89. Answer A

- Hematology Section: This department deals with the handling of various blood specimens. Tests performed in this department include WBC counts, RBC counts, hemoglobin, hematocrit (Hct), RBC indices, and platelet counts. The results of these tests indicate conditions such as dehydration, anemia, leukemia, and a wide variety of other diseases.

90. Answer C

- WBC counts, RBC counts, hemoglobin, hematocrit (Hct), RBC indices, and platelet counts: These are the tests commonly performed in the Hematology Section.

91. Answer C

- Dehydration, anemia, leukemia, and a wide variety of other diseases: The results of tests performed in the Hematology Section indicate conditions such as dehydration, anemia, leukemia, and a wide variety of other diseases.

92. Answer B

- Chemistry Section: This is the department in the medical laboratory that performs tests for blood glucose levels, electrolytes (sodium, potassium, chloride), total protein, etc.

93. Answer C

- Presence of a liver disorder: The results of tests performed in the Chemistry Section can indicate the presence of a liver disorder.

94. Answer C

- Blood Bank Section: This is the section of the laboratory where blood is collected, stored, and prepared for transfusion.

95. Answer A

- Standards for patient identification and specimen handling: It is essential for all staff members to comply with the standards for patient identification and specimen handling in the Blood Bank Section in order to ensure the safety of all the patients.

96. Answer C

- Electrolytes (sodium, potassium, chloride): Electrolytes are not commonly tested in the Hematology Section.

97. Answer C

- Blood type and compatibility for transfusion: The results of tests performed in the Blood Bank Section indicate the blood type and compatibility for transfusion.

98. Answer D

- Anatomical Pathology Section: This section of the laboratory deals with surgical and anatomical pathology analysis.

99. Answer C

- Blood glucose levels, electrolytes (sodium, potassium, chloride), total protein, etc.: These are the tests commonly performed in the Chemistry Section.

100. Answer C

- To handle various blood specimens and perform tests for conditions such as dehydration, anemia, leukemia, and a wide variety of other diseases: The purpose of the Hematology Section in the medical laboratory is to handle various blood specimens and perform tests for conditions such as dehydration, anemia, leukemia, and a wide variety of other diseases.

MEDICAL ASSISTANT CERTIFICATION
EXAMINATION STUDY GUIDE
PART-TWO

1. What is the primary goal of the health care system?

    a. To provide affordable care to all citizens

    b. To provide high-quality care to all citizens

    c. To provide care to only those who can afford it.

    d. To provide care to only those who are insured.

2. Which of the following is not a type of health care system?

    a. Single-payer system

    b. Multi-payer system

    c. Private system

    d. Social system

3. Which of the following is a disadvantage of a single-payer health care system?

    a. Limited access to care

    b. High administrative costs

    c. Limited choice of providers

    d. High out-of-pocket costs

4. Which of the following is a disadvantage of a multi-payer health care system?

    a. Limited access to care

    b. High administrative costs

    c. Limited choice of providers

    d. High out-of-pocket costs

5. Which of the following is a disadvantage of a private health care system?

    a. Limited access to care

    b. High administrative costs

    c. Limited choice of providers

    d. High out-of-pocket costs

6. Which of the following is a disadvantage of a social health care system?

    a. Limited access to care

    b. High administrative costs

    c. Limited choice of providers

    d. High out-of-pocket costs

7. Which of the following is a characteristic of a single-payer health care system?

    a. Multiple insurance companies

    b. Government-funded health care

    c. Private insurance companies

    d. Employer-funded health care

8. Which of the following is a characteristic of a multi-payer health care system?

    a. Government-funded health care

    b. Private insurance companies

    c. Employer-funded health care

    d. No insurance companies.

9. Which of the following is a characteristic of a private health care system?

   a. Government-funded health care

   b. Private insurance companies

   c. Employer-funded health care

   d. No insurance companies.

10. Which of the following is a characteristic of a social health care system?

   a. Government-funded health care

   b. Private insurance companies

   c. Employer-funded health care

   d. No insurance companies.

11. Which of the following is a benefit of a single-payer health care system?

   a. Increased choice of providers

   b. Lower administrative costs

   c. Lower out-of-pocket costs

   d. Increased competition among insurance companies

12. Which of the following is a benefit of a multi-payer health care system?

   a. Increased choice of providers

   b. Lower administrative costs

   c. Lower out-of-pocket costs

   d. Increased competition among insurance companies

13. Which of the following is a benefit of a private health care system?

    a.   Increased choice of providers

    b.   Lower administrative costs

    c.   Lower out-of-pocket costs

    d.   Increased competition among insurance companies

14. Which of the following is a benefit of a social health care system?

    a.   Increased choice of providers

    b.   Lower administrative costs

    c.   Lower out-of-pocket costs

    d.   Increased competition among insurance companies

15. Which of the following is a reason why health care costs are rising in the United States?

    a.   Increased competition among insurance companies

    b.   Increased use of preventive care

    c.   Increased use of technology

    d.   Decreased use of prescription drugs

16. Which of the following is a reason why health care costs are lower in other countries?

    a.   Lower use of technology

    b.   Lower use of preventive care

    c.   Higher use of prescription drugs

    d.   Higher administrative costs

17. Which of the following is a reason why the United States has a higher infant mortality rate than other developed countries?

    a.   Lack of access to health care

    b.   Higher use of technology

    c.   Higher use of preventive care

    d.   Higher use of prescription drugs

18. Which of the following is a reason why the United States spends more on health care than other developed countries?

    a.   Higher use of preventive care

    b.   Higher use of prescription drugs

    c.   Lower use of technology

    d.   Lower administrative costs

19. Which of the following is a reason why the United States has a higher rate of medical errors compared to other developed countries?

    a.   Lack of access to health care

    b.   Higher use of technology

    c.   Higher use of preventive care

    d.   Higher use of prescription drugs

20. Which of the following is a reason why the United States has a higher rate of chronic diseases compared to other developed countries?

    a. Lack of access to health care

    b. Higher use of technology

    c. Higher use of preventive care

    d. Higher use of prescription drugs

21. Which of the following is a reason why the United States has a higher rate of obesity compared to other developed countries?

    a. Lack of access to health care

    b. Higher use of technology

    c. Higher use of preventive care

    d. Higher use of prescription drugs

22. Which of the following is a reason why the United States has a higher rate of mental health disorders compared to other developed countries?

    a. Lack of access to health care

    b. Higher use of technology

    c. Higher use of preventive care

    d. Higher use of prescription drugs

23. Which of the following is a reason why the United States has a higher rate of medical bankruptcy compared to other developed countries?

    a. Lack of access to health care

    b. Higher use of technology

    c. Higher use of preventive care

    d. Higher use of prescription drugs

24. Which of the following is a reason why the United States has a higher rate of uninsured individuals compared to other developed countries?

    a. Lack of access to health care

    b. Higher use of technology

    c. Higher use of preventive care

    d. Higher use of prescription drugs

25. Which of the following is a reason why the United States has a higher rate of health care-related lawsuits compared to other developed countries?

    a. Lack of access to health care

    b. Higher use of technology

    c. Higher use of preventive care

    d. Higher use of prescription drugs

26. Which of the following is a reason why the United States has a higher rate of prescription drug costs compared to other developed countries?

    a. Lack of access to health care

    b. Higher use of technology

    c. Higher use of preventive care

    d. Higher use of prescription drugs

27. Which of the following is a reason why the United States has a higher rate of administrative costs compared to other developed countries?

    a. Lack of access to health care

    b. Higher use of technology

    c. Higher use of preventive care

    d. Higher use of prescription drugs

28. Which of the following is a reason why the United States has a higher rate of health care spending compared to other developed countries?

    a. Lack of access to health care

    b. Higher use of technology

    c. Higher use of preventive care

    d. Higher use of prescription drugs

29. Which of the following is a reason why the United States has a higher rate of hospital readmissions compared to other developed countries?

    a. Lack of access to health care

    b. Higher use of technology

    c. Higher use of preventive care

    d. Higher use of prescription drugs

30. Which of the following is a reason why the United States has a higher rate of emergency room visits compared to other developed countries?

    a. Lack of access to health care

    b. Higher use of technology

    c. Higher use of preventive care

    d. Higher use of prescription drugs

31. Which of the following is a reason why the United States has a higher rate of medical imaging tests compared to other developed countries?

    a. Lack of access to health care

    b. Higher use of technology

    c. Higher use of preventive care

    d. Higher use of prescription drugs

32. Which of the following is the most effective way to prevent the spread of infection?

    a. Wearing gloves

    b. Washing hands

    c. Wearing a mask

    d. Using hand sanitizer

33. Which of the following is an example of a bloodborne pathogen?

    a. Influenza virus

    b. Hepatitis B virus

    c. Staphylococcus aureus

    d. Streptococcus pneumoniae

34. Which of the following is an example of a contact transmission route for infection?

    a. Coughing and sneezing

    b. Touching contaminated surfaces

    c. Inhaling droplets from an infected person

    d. Being bitten by an infected animal

35. Which of the following is an example of a droplet transmission route for infection?

   a. Coughing and sneezing

   b. Touching contaminated surfaces

   c. Inhaling droplets from an infected person

   d. Being bitten by an infected animal

36. Which of the following is an example of an airborne transmission route for infection?

   a. Coughing and sneezing

   b. Touching contaminated surfaces

   c. Inhaling droplets from an infected person

   d. Being bitten by an infected animal

37. Which of the following is an example of a vector-borne transmission route for infection?

   a. Coughing and sneezing

   b. Touching contaminated surfaces

   c. Inhaling droplets from an infected person

   d. Being bitten by an infected animal

38. Which of the following is an example of a fomite transmission route for infection?

   a. Coughing and sneezing

   b. Touching contaminated surfaces

   c. Inhaling droplets from an infected person

   d. Being bitten by an infected animal

39. Which of the following is an example of a nosocomial infection?

   a. Influenza virus

   b. Hepatitis B virus

   c. Staphylococcus aureus

   d. Streptococcus pneumoniae

40. Which of the following is an example of a community-acquired infection?

   a. Influenza virus

   b. Hepatitis B virus

   c. Staphylococcus aureus

   d. Streptococcus pneumoniae

41. Which of the following is an example of a healthcare-associated infection?

   a. Influenza virus

   b. Hepatitis B virus

   c. Staphylococcus aureus

   d. Streptococcus pneumoniae

42. Which of the following is an example of a multidrug-resistant organism?

   a. Influenza virus

   b. Hepatitis B virus

   c. Methicillin-resistant Staphylococcus aureus (MRSA)

   d. Streptococcus pneumoniae

43. Which of the following is an example of personal protective equipment (PPE)?

    a. Hand sanitizer

    b. Gloves

    c. Soap

    d. Disinfectant spray

44. Which of the following is an example of a standard precaution for infection control?

    a. Wearing gloves

    b. Wearing a mask

    c. Using hand sanitizer

    d. Washing hands

45. Which of the following is an example of a transmission-based precaution for infection control?

    a. Wearing gloves

    b. Wearing a mask

    c. Using hand sanitizer

    d. Washing hands

46. Which of the following is an example of a sharp injury?

    a. A cut from a contaminated object

    b. A burn from a hot surface

    c. A sprain from a fall

    d. A bruise from a blunt force

47. Which of the following is an example of a chemical exposure in the healthcare setting?

   a. Exposure to bloodborne pathogens

   b. Exposure to radiation

   c. Exposure to hazardous drugs

   d. Exposure to infectious diseases

48. Which of the following is an example of radiation exposure in a healthcare setting?

   a. Exposure to bloodborne pathogens

   b. Exposure to chemicals

   c. Exposure to hazardous drugs

   d. Exposure to X-rays

49. Which of the following is an example of a fire hazard in a healthcare setting?

   a. Improper disposal of hazardous waste

   b. Overcrowding in patient rooms

   c. Use of flammable liquids

   d. Lack of hand hygiene

50. Which of the following is an example of an electrical hazard in the healthcare setting?

   a. Improper disposal of hazardous waste

   b. Overcrowding in patient rooms

   c. Use of flammable liquids

   d. Use of damaged electrical equipment

51. Which of the following is an example of a physical hazard in the healthcare setting?

    a. Exposure to bloodborne pathogens

    b. Exposure to chemicals

    c. Exposure to hazardous drugs

    d. Slip, trip, and fall hazards.

52. Which of the following is an example of a biological hazard in the healthcare setting?

    a. Exposure to radiation

    b. Exposure to chemicals

    c. Exposure to infectious diseases

    d. Exposure to noise

53. Which of the following is an example of a mechanical hazard in the healthcare setting?

    a. Exposure to bloodborne pathogens

    b. Exposure to chemicals

    c. Exposure to hazardous drugs

    d. Use of malfunctioning equipment

54. Which of the following is an example of a patient safety event?

    a. Medication error

    b. Exposure to hazardous waste

    c. Fire hazard

    d. Electrical hazard

55. Which of the following is an example of a near miss in patient safety?

    a. A patient falls and sustains an injury.

    b. A medication error is caught before it reaches the patient.

    c. A fire broke out in a patient's room.

    d. A patient is exposed to hazardous waste.

56. Which of the following is an example of a root cause analysis in patient safety?

    a. Identifying the cause of a medication error

    b. Identifying the cause of a fire hazard

    c. Identifying the cause of a slip, trip, and fall hazard.

    d. Identifying the cause of a biological hazard

57. Which of the following is an example of a failure mode and effects analysis in patient safety?

    a. Identifying the cause of a medication error

    b. Identifying the cause of a fire hazard

    c. Identifying the cause of a slip, trip, and fall hazard.

    d. Identifying the potential failure modes of a medical device

58. Which of the following is an example of a just culture in patient safety?

    a. Blaming and punishing individuals for errors

    b. Encouraging reporting of errors and near misses

    c. Ignoring errors and near misses

    d. Focusing on individual performance rather than system issues

59. Which of the following is an example of a high-reliability organization in patient safety?

    a. A hospital with a high rate of medication errors

    b. A hospital with a high rate of patient falls

    c. A hospital with a culture of safety and a low rate of adverse events

    d. A hospital with a culture of blame and punishment

60. Which of the following is an example of a safety culture in healthcare?

    a. A culture of blame and punishment

    b. A culture of fear and intimidation

    c. A culture of transparency and accountability

    d. A culture of individual performance rather than system issues

61. Which of the following is an example of a safety event reporting system in healthcare?

    a. A system that punishes individuals for errors

    b. A system that encourages reporting of errors and near misses

    c. A system that ignores errors and near misses

    d. A system that focuses on individual performance rather than system issues

62. Which of the following is an example of a safety checklist in healthcare?

    a. A list of punishments for errors

    b. A list of individual performance metrics

    c. A list of system issues to be addressed.

    d. A list of steps to be followed to ensure patient safety.

63. Which body cavity houses the lungs, heart, esophagus, and trachea?

    a. Cranial cavity

    b. Spinal cavity

    c. Thoracic cavity

    d. Abdominopelvic cavity

64. Which region of the abdomen is located on the right side and just below the ribs?

    a. Epigastric region

    b. Right hypochondriac region

    c. Right lumbar region

    d. Right iliac (inguinal) region

65. Which type of molecule is used for energy production and can be found in butter and oils?

    a. Carbohydrates

    b. Lipids

    c. Proteins

    d. Nucleic acids

66. Which type of molecule is used to make cell membranes?

    a. Carbohydrates

    b. Lipids

    c. Proteins

    d. Nucleic acids

67. Which type of molecule is the building block of tissues?

    a.   Carbohydrates

    b.   Lipids

    c.   Proteins

    d.   Nucleic acids

68. Which type of molecule contains the genetic recipe of life?

    a.   Carbohydrates

    b.   Lipids

    c.   Proteins

    d.   Nucleic acids

69. Which quadrant of the abdomen is located on the left side and just below the ribs?

    a.   Left hypochondriac region.

    b.   Left lumbar region.

    c.   Left iliac (inguinal) region.

    d.   Hypogastric region

70. What is an organ?

    a.   A collection of similar cells acting together to perform a function.

    b.   The smallest structural unit of the nervous system

    c.   A layer of tissue that lines body cavities, covers organs, and separates structures.

    d.   An imaginary plane used as a reference in describing positions.

71. What is a tissue?

    a.   A collection of similar cells acting together to perform a function.

    b.   The smallest structural unit of the nervous system

    c.   A layer of tissue that lines body cavities, covers organs, and separates structures.

    d.   An imaginary plane used as a reference in describing positions.

72. What is a neuron?

    a.   A collection of similar cells acting together to perform a function.

    b.   The smallest structural unit of the nervous system

    c.   A layer of tissue that lines body cavities, covers organs, and separates structures.

    d.   An imaginary plane used as a reference in describing positions.

73. What is a nephron?

    a.   A collection of similar cells acting together to perform a function.

    b.   The smallest structural unit of the nervous system

    c.   The functional unit of the kidney

    d.   An imaginary plane used as a reference in describing positions.

74. What is the function of mitochondria?

    a.   To provide protection

    b.   To regulate body temperature

    c.   To serve as a function for cellular respiration

    d.   To synthesize vitamin D

75. What is a membrane?

    a. A collection of similar cells acting together to perform a function.

    b. The smallest structural unit of the nervous system

    c. A layer of tissue that lines body cavities, covers organs, and separates structures.

    d. An imaginary plane used as a reference in describing positions.

76. What is the frontal plane?

    a. A plane that divides the body into front and back halves

    b. A plane that divides the body into left and right portions

    c. A plane that passes along the midline and divides the body into equal left and right halves.

    d. A plane that divides the body into upper and lower halves

77. What is the midsagittal plane?

    a. A plane that divides the body into front and back halves

    b. A plane that divides the body into left and right portions

    c. A plane that passes along the midline and divides the body into equal left and right halves.

    d. A plane that divides the body into upper and lower halves

78. What is the function of the integumentary system?

    a. To provide protection

    b. To regulate body temperature

    c. To provide sensory reception

    d. All of the above

79. What is the main function of the skin?

    a. To provide protection

    b. To regulate body temperature

    c. To provide sensory reception

    d. All of the above

80. What is the liquid portion of the blood in its anticoagulated state?

    a. Serum

    b. Plasma

    c. Hemoglobin

    d. Thrombocytes

81. What is the pigment responsible for the reddish color of the blood?

    a. Hemoglobin

    b. Serum

    c. Plasma

    d. Thrombocytes

82. Which type of white blood cells defend the body against infectious diseases?

    a. Neutrophils

    b. Lymphocytes

    c. Monocytes

    d. Eosinophils

83. What is the function of platelets in the blood?

    a. To provide support in cell-mediated immunity

    b. To aid in allergic or inflammatory responses

    c. To form blood clots when a blood vessel is damaged.

    d. To provide a boost to immune defense of the body

84. What is the average amount of blood within the body of the average human adult?

    a. 1-2 liters

    b. 3-4 liters

    c. 5-6 liters

    d. 7-8 liters

85. What is the muscular organ that acts as the pump for the circulatory system?

    a. Lungs

    b. Liver

    c. Heart

    d. Kidneys

86. What is the function of the respiratory system?

    a. To provide oxygen to cells and remove carbon dioxide from them.

    b. To change food so that it can be used in the body.

    c. To coordinate many body functions through hormone secretions

    d. To return excess interstitial fluid to the blood and help protect the body against disease.

87. What is the digestive tract?

    a.   The wall of the digestive system

    b.   The organs of the respiratory system

    c.   The organs of the circulatory system

    d.   The organs of the endocrine system

88. What is the function of the endocrine system?

    a.   To provide oxygen to cells and remove carbon dioxide from them.

    b.   To change food so that it can be used in the body.

    c.   To coordinate many body functions through hormone secretions

    d.   To return excess interstitial fluid to the blood and help protect the body against disease.

89. What is the layer of the heart that is responsible for pumping blood?

    a.   Epicardium

    b.   Myocardium

    c.   Endocardium

    d.   Lymphatic layer

90. What is myopia?

    a.   A severe form of farsightedness

    b.   A clouding of a normally clear lens of the eye

    c.   A severe form of nearsightedness

    d.   An irregular focusing of the light rays entering the eye.

91. What is hyperopia?

    a.   A severe form of farsightedness

    b.   A clouding of a normally clear lens of the eye

    c.   A severe form of nearsightedness

    d.   An irregular focusing of the light rays entering the eye.

92. What is presbyopia?

    a.   A severe form of farsightedness

    b.   A clouding of a normally clear lens of the eye

    c.   Inability to focus with the lens because of loss of its elasticity.

    d.   An irregular focusing of the light rays entering the eye.

93. What is astigmatism?

    a.   A severe form of farsightedness

    b.   A clouding of a normally clear lens of the eye

    c.   A severe form of nearsightedness

    d.   An irregular focusing of the light rays entering the eye.

94. What is strabismus?

    a.   A clouding of a normally clear lens of the eye

    b.   An irregular focusing of the light rays entering the eye.

    c.   Disorder in which the visual axes of the eyes are not directed at the same point.

    d.   A severe form of nearsightedness

95. What is cataract?

    a. A clouding of a normally clear lens of the eye

    b. A severe form of farsightedness

    c. A severe form of nearsightedness

    d. An irregular focusing of the light rays entering the eye.

96. What is glaucoma?

    a. A clouding of a normally clear lens of the eye

    b. A severe form of farsightedness

    c. A severe form of nearsightedness

    d. Increased intraocular pressure, which can result in damage to the optic nerve.

97. What is retinal detachment?

    a. An infection of the ear canal

    b. Total hearing loss

    c. Elevation of the retina from the choroid

    d. Dizziness

98. What is otalgia?

    a. Total hearing loss

    b. Dizziness

    c. Earache

    d. Infection of the middle ear

99. What is external otitis?

    a. painful urination

    b. Total hearing loss

    c. Swimmer's ear; an infection of the ear canal

    d. All

100. What is urinary tract infection (UTI)?

    a. Involuntary discharge of urine, most often due to lack of bladder control

    b. Painful urination

    c. Bacteria or any other organism that can be found in the urethra or ureter that cause painful urination and malaise.

    d. Total hearing loss

PART –TWO

ANSWER TO MEDICAL ASSISTANT EXAM QUESTIONS

1. **Answer: B**

    The primary goal of the health care system is to provide high-quality care to all citizens.

2. **Answer: D**

    The social system is not a type of health care system. The other three options are types of health care systems.

3. **Answer: A**

    Limited access to care is a disadvantage of a single-payer health care system.

4. **Answer: B**

    High administrative costs are a disadvantage of a multi-payer health care system.

5. **Answer: A**

    Limited access to care is a disadvantage of a private health care system.

6. **Answer: C**

    Limited choice of providers is a disadvantage of a social health care system.

7. **Answer: B**

    Government-funded health care is a characteristic of a single-payer health care system.

8. **Answer: B**

    Private insurance companies are a characteristic of a multi-payer health care system.

9. **Answer: B**

    Private insurance companies are a characteristic of a private health care system.

10. **Answer: A**

    Government-funded health care is a characteristic of a social health care system.

11. **Answer: B**

Lower administrative costs are a benefit of a single-payer health care system.

12. **Answer: A**

Increased choice of providers is a benefit of a multi-payer health care system.

13. **Answer: A**

Increased choice of providers is a benefit of a private health care system.

14. **Answer: C**

Lower out-of-pocket costs are a benefit of a social health care system.

15. **Answer: C**

Increased use of technology is a reason why health care costs are rising in the United States.

16. **Answer: A**

Lower use of technology is a reason why health care costs are lower in other countries.

17. **Answer: A**

Lack of access to health care is a reason why the United States has a higher infant mortality rate than other developed countries.

18. **Answer: B**

Higher use of prescription drugs is a reason why the United States spends more on health care than other developed countries.

19. **Answer: B**

Higher use of technology is a reason why the United States has a higher rate of medical errors compared to other developed countries.

20. **Answer: A**

Lack of access to health care is a reason why the United States has a higher rate of chronic diseases compared to other developed countries.

21. Answer: A

Lack of access to health care is a reason why the United States has a higher rate of obesity compared to other developed countries.

22. Answer: A

Lack of access to health care is a reason why the United States has a higher rate of mental health disorders compared to other developed countries.

23. Answer: A

Lack of access to health care is a reason why the United States has a higher rate of medical bankruptcy compared to other developed countries.

24. Answer: A

Lack of access to health care is a reason why the United States has a higher rate of uninsured individuals compared to other developed countries.

25. Answer: B

Higher use of technology is a reason why the United States has a higher rate of health care-related lawsuits compared to other developed countries.

26. Answer: D

Higher use of prescription drugs is a reason why the United States has a higher rate of prescription drug costs compared to other developed countries.

27. Answer: D

Higher use of prescription drugs is not a reason why the United States has a higher rate of administrative costs compared to other developed countries.

28. Answer: B

Higher use of technology is a reason why the United States has a higher rate of health care spending compared to other developed countries.

29. Answer: A

Lack of access to health care is a reason why the United States has a higher rate of hospital readmissions compared to other developed countries.

30. **Answer: A**

Lack of access to health care is a reason why the United States has a higher rate of emergency room visits compared to other developed countries.

31. **Answer: B**

Higher use of technology is a reason why the United States has a higher rate of medical imaging tests compared to other developed countries.

32. **Answer: B**

Washing hands is the most effective way to prevent the spread of infection as it removes dirt, germs, and bacteria from the hands.

33. **Answer: B**

Bloodborne pathogens are infectious microorganisms that can be transmitted through blood and other bodily fluids.

34. **Answer: B**

Contact transmission occurs when an individual comes into contact with a contaminated surface or object.

35. **Answer: C**

Droplet transmission occurs when an individual inhales droplets from an infected persons cough or sneeze.

36. **Answer: A**

Airborne transmission occurs when an individual inhales small particles or droplets that are suspended in the air.

37. **Answer: D**

Vector-borne transmission occurs when an individual is bitten by an infected animal, such as a mosquito or tick.

38. Answer: B

Fomite transmission occurs when an individual comes into contact with a contaminated object or surface.

39. Answer: C

Nosocomial infections are infections that are acquired in a healthcare setting.

40. Answer: A

Community-acquired infections are infections that are acquired outside of a healthcare setting.

41. Answer: B

Healthcare-associated infections are infections that are acquired in a healthcare setting.

42. Answer: C

Multidrug-resistant organisms are microorganisms that are resistant to multiple antibiotics.

43. Answer: B

Personal protective equipment (PPE) is equipment worn to minimize exposure to hazards that can cause serious workplace injuries and illnesses.

44. Answer: D

Standard precautions are basic infection prevention measures that should be used with all patients to prevent the spread of infection.

45. Answer: B

Transmission-based precautions are additional precautions used when an individual is known or suspected to be infected with a highly infectious agent.

46. Answer: A

A sharps injury is a puncture wound or cut caused by a contaminated object, such as a needle or scalpel.

47. Answer: C

Chemical exposure occurs when an individual is exposed to hazardous chemicals, such as chemotherapy drugs.

48. Answer: D

Radiation exposure occurs when an individual is exposed to ionizing radiation, such as X-rays.

49. Answer: C

Fire hazards in the healthcare setting can be caused by the use of flammable liquids, such as alcohol-based hand sanitizers.

50. Answer: D

Electrical hazards in the healthcare setting can be caused by the use of damaged electrical equipment.

51. Answer: D

Physical hazards in the healthcare setting can include slip, trip, and fall hazards.

52. Answer: C

Biological hazards in the healthcare setting can include exposure to infectious diseases.

53. Answer: D

Mechanical hazards in the healthcare setting can include the use of malfunctioning equipment.

54. Answer: A

A patient safety event is any event or circumstance that could have resulted or did result in harm to a patient.

55. Answer: B

A near miss in patient safety is an event or circumstance that could have resulted in harm to a patient but did not.

56. Answer: A

Root cause analysis is a process used to identify the underlying cause of an event or problem.

57. Answer: D

Failure mode and effects analysis is a process used to identify potential failure modes of a system or process and their effects.

58. Answer: B

Just culture is a culture that encourages reporting of errors and near misses and focuses on system issues rather than individual blame.

59. Answer: C

High-reliability organizations are organizations that have a culture of safety and a low rate of adverse events.

60. Answer: C

Safety culture in healthcare is a culture that values transparency, accountability, and a focus on patient safety.

61. Answer: B

Safety event reporting systems are systems that encourage reporting of safety events and near misses to improve patient safety.

62. Answer: D

Safety checklists are lists of steps to be followed to ensure patient safety and prevent errors.

63. Answer C

Thoracic cavity: The body cavity that houses the lungs, heart, esophagus, and trachea.

64. Answer B

Right hypochondriac region: The region of the abdomen located on the right side and just below the ribs.

65. Answer B

Lipids

A type of molecule used for energy production and can be found in butter and oils.

66. Answer B

Lipids

A type of molecule used to make cell membranes.

67. Answer C

Proteins

The building block of tissues.

68. Answer D

Nucleic acid

: A type of molecule that contains the genetic recipe of life.

69. Answer A

Left hypochondriac region.

The region of the abdomen is located on the left side and just below the ribs.

70. Answer A

Organ: A collection of similar cells acting together to perform a function

A structure that is composed of two or more tissue types and performs a specific function in the body.

71. Answer A

Tissue:

A collection of similar cells that work together to perform a specific function in the body.

72. Answer B

Neuron:

The smallest structural unit of the nervous system, consisting of a cell body, dendrites, and an axon.

73. Answer C

Nephron:

functional unit of the kidney, responsible for filtering blood and producing urine.

74. Answer C

Mitochondria: To serve as a function for cellular respiration

Organelles found in cells are responsible for producing energy through cellular respiration.

75. Answer C

Membrane:

A layer of tissue that lines body cavities, covers organs, and separates structures.

76. Answer A

Frontal plane:

An imaginary plane that divides the body into front and back halves.

77. Answer C

Midsagittal plane:

An imaginary plane that passes along the midline and divides the body into equal left and right halves.

78. Answer D

Integumentary system:

The system that includes the skin and its derivatives, such as hair, nails, and glands, and is responsible for protecting the body, regulating body temperature, and providing sensory reception.

79. Answer D

Skin:

The largest organ of the body, responsible for protecting the body from external damage, regulating body temperature, and providing sensory reception.

80. **Answer: B**

Plasma - Plasma is the liquid portion of the blood in its anticoagulated (or unclothed) state, accounting for 55 to 65 percent of the blood volume.

81. Answer: A

Hemoglobin - Hemoglobin is the pigment responsible for the reddish color of the blood. It is found in red blood cells and is responsible for carrying oxygen from the lungs to the body's tissues.

82. **Answer: A**

Neutrophils - Neutrophils are the most common type of white blood cells and defend the body against infectious diseases by engulfing and destroying bacteria and other foreign invaders.

83. **Answer: C**

To form blood clots when a blood vessel is damaged - Platelets, also known as thrombocytes, are the smallest cells found in the blood and aid in the process of coagulation, the formation of blood clots that occurs when a blood vessel is damaged.

84. **Answer: C**

5-6 liters - The amount of blood within the body of the average human adult is equivalent to a measurement of five or six liters.

85. **Answer: C**

Heart - The heart is the muscular organ that acts as the pump for the circulatory system.

86. **Answer: A**

To provide oxygen to cells and remove carbon dioxide from them - The respiratory system is responsible for providing oxygen to cells and helps remove carbon dioxide from them.

87. **Answer: A**

The wall of the digestive system - The digestive tract runs from the mouth to the anus and consists of four layers or tunics, the mucosa, submucosa, the muscular layer, and the serous layer or serosa.

88. **Answer: C**

To coordinate many body functions through hormone secretions - The endocrine system consists of glands whose secretions coordinate many body functions. The glands are ductless glands that secrete hormones directly into the bloodstream.

89. **Answer: B**

Myocardium - The myocardium is the middle layer of the heart and is responsible for pumping blood.

90. **Answer: C**

A severe form of nearsightedness - Myopia is a vision condition in which people can see close objects clearly, but objects farther away appear blurred.

91. **Answer: A**

A severe form of farsightedness - Hyperopia is a vision condition in which people can see distant objects clearly, but objects up close appear blurred.

92. **Answer: C**

Inability to focus with the lens because of loss of its elasticity - Presbyopia is a vision condition in which the lens of the eye loses its flexibility, making it difficult to focus on close objects.

93. **Answer: D**

An irregular focusing of the light rays entering the eye - Astigmatism is a vision condition in which the cornea or lens of the eye is irregularly shaped, causing blurred or distorted vision.

94. **Answer: C**

a. Disorder in which the visual axes of the eyes are not directed at the same point - Strabismus is a vision condition in which the eyes are not aligned properly and do not work together to focus on an object.

95. **Answer: A**

A clouding of a normally clear lens of the eye - Cataract is a vision condition in which the lens of the eye becomes cloudy, causing vision loss.

96. **Answer: D**

Increased intraocular pressure, which can result in damage to the optic nerve - Glaucoma is a group of eye diseases that cause damage to the optic nerve and can lead to vision loss or blindness.

97. **Answer: C**

Elevation of the retina from the choroid - Retinal detachment is a vision condition in which the retina separates from the underlying tissue, causing vision loss.

98. **Answer: C**

Earache - Otalgia is a medical term for earache, which is pain in the ear.

99. **Answer: C**

Swimmer's ear: an infection of the ear canal - External otitis, also known as swimmer's ear, is an infection of the ear canal that can cause pain, itching, and swelling.

100. **Answer: C**

Bacteria or any other organism that can be found in the urethra or ureter that cause painful urination and malaise - Urinary tract infection (UTI) is an infection caused by bacteria or other organisms in the urinary tract, which can cause painful urination and other symptoms.

MEDICAL ASSISTANT CERTIFICATION
EXAMINATION STUDY GUIDE
PART-THREE

1. What is gonorrhea?

    a. A serious sexually transmitted disease

    b. A condition that causes cessation of menstrual periods

    c. An inflammation and infection of the vaginal tissues

    d. An inflammation of the genital mucous membrane of male and female

2. What is syphilis?

    a. A serious sexually transmitted disease

    b. A condition that causes cessation of menstrual periods

    c. An inflammation and infection of the vaginal tissues

    d. An inflammation of the genital mucous membrane of male and female

3. How is HIV transferred?

    a. By direct sexual contact

    b. By contaminated food and water

    c. By inhaling contaminated air

    d. By physical contact with an infected person

4. What is the diagnosis for HIV?

    a. A urine tests.

    b. A blood tests.

    c. A saliva tests.

    d. A skin tests.

5. What is AIDS?

    a. A serious sexually transmitted disease

    b. A condition that causes cessation of menstrual periods

    c. A result of the HIV virus

    d. An inflammation and infection of the vaginal tissues

6. What is pelvic inflammatory disease?

    a. An inflammation and infection of the vaginal tissues

    b. A condition that causes cessation of menstrual periods

    c. Inflammation and serious infection of organs in the pelvic cavity

    d. An inflammation of the genital mucous membrane of male and female

7. What is vaginitis?

    a. An inflammation and infection of the vaginal tissues

    b. A condition that causes cessation of menstrual periods

    c. Inflammation and serious infection of organs in the pelvic cavity

    d. An inflammation of the genital mucous membrane of male and female

8. What is menopause?

    a. An inflammation and infection of the vaginal tissues

    b. A condition that causes cessation of menstrual periods

    c. Inflammation and serious infection of organs in the pelvic cavity

    d. An inflammation of the genital mucous membrane of male and female

9. What is the average duration of the chronic asymptomatic or latency phase of AIDS?

    a. A few days

    b. 1-2 years

    c. 5-7 years

    d. 10 years

10. What is the ultimate result of the HIV virus?

   a. Gonorrhea

   b. Syphilis

   c. Pelvic inflammatory disease

   d. AIDS

11. What is the most common cause of pelvic inflammatory disease?

   a. Pregnancy

   b. Menopause

   c. Sexual activity

   d. Aging

12. What is the characteristic symptom of vaginitis?

   a. Cessation of menstrual periods

   b. Inflammation and infection of the vaginal tissues

   c. Foul-smelling vaginal discharge

   d. Inflammation of the genital mucous membrane of male and female

13. What is the primary symptom of gonorrhea?

   a. Cessation of menstrual periods

   b. Inflammation and infection of the vaginal tissues

   c. Foul-smelling vaginal discharge

   d. Inflammation of the genital mucous membrane of male and female

14. What is the primary symptom of syphilis?

   a. Cessation of menstrual periods

   b. Inflammation and infection of the vaginal tissues

   c. Foul-smelling vaginal discharge

   d. Sores or rash on the genitals or mouth

15. What is the primary mode of transmission for HIV?

   a. Sexual contact

   b. Sharing food and drinks

   c. Touching an infected person

   d. Breathing contaminated air

16. What is the primary symptoms of menopause?

   a. Inflammation and infection of the vaginal tissues

   b. Foul-smelling vaginal discharge

   c. Cessation of menstrual periods

   d. Inflammation of the genital mucous membrane of male and female

17. What are the primary symptoms of chronic asymptomatic or latency phase of AIDS?

   a. Sores or rash on the genitals or mouth

   b. Foul smelling vaginal discharge

   c. Cessation of menstrual periods

   d. No symptoms are present.

18. What is the primary symptom of the AIDS phase?

   a. Inflammation and infection of the vaginal tissues

   b. Foul-smelling vaginal discharge

   c. Cessation of menstrual periods

   d. Opportunistic infections that would otherwise be eliminated by a healthy individual's immune response.

19. What is the primary mode of transmission for syphilis?

   a. Sexual contact

   b. Sharing food and drinks

   c. Touching an infected person

   d. Breathing contaminated air

20. What is the primary symptom of pelvic inflammatory disease?

    a. Inflammation and infection of the vaginal tissues

    b. Foul-smelling vaginal discharge

    c. Pain in the lower abdomen

    d. Inflammation of the genital mucous membrane of male and female

21. What is fibroadenoma?

    a. A painful menstrual period

    b. A benign tumor of the breast

    c. Proliferation of endometrial tissue outside of the uterus

    d. Implantation of the fertilized ovum outside the uterus

22. What is amenorrhea?

    a. Painful menstruation

    b. Absence of menstruation at puberty

    c. Proliferation of endometrial tissue outside of the uterus

    d. Implantation of the fertilized ovum outside the uterus

23. What is endometriosis?

    a. A painful menstrual period

    b. A benign tumor of the breast

    c. Proliferation of endometrial tissue outside of the uterus

    d. Implantation of the fertilized ovum outside the uterus

24. What is ectopic pregnancy?

    a. A painful menstrual period

    b. A benign tumor of the breast

    c. Proliferation of endometrial tissue outside of the uterus

    d. Implantation of the fertilized ovum outside the uterus

25. What is miscarriage?

    a.   A painful menstrual period

    b.   A benign tumor of the breast

    c.   Spontaneous abortion

    d.   Implantation of the fertilized ovum outside the uterus

26. What is placenta previa?

    a.   A painful menstrual period

    b.   A benign tumor of the breast

    c.   Proliferation of endometrial tissue outside of the uterus

    d.   Implantation of the placenta in the lower uterine segment on the internal cervical lining

27. What is orchitis?

    a.   Infection of the testes caused by viral or bacterial infection or injury.

    b.   Acute or chronic inflammation of the prostate gland

    c.   Failure to initiate or maintain an erection.

    d.   Enlargement of the prostate gland

28. What is prostatitis?

    a.   Infection of the testes caused by viral or bacterial infection or injury.

    b.   Acute or chronic inflammation of the prostate gland

    c.   Failure to initiate or maintain an erection.

    d.   Enlargement of the prostate gland

29. What is impotence?

    a.   Infection of the testes caused by viral or bacterial infection or injury.

    b.   Acute or chronic inflammation of the prostate gland

    c.   Failure to initiate or maintain an erection.

    d.   Enlargement of the prostate gland

30. What is benign prostatic hyperplasia?

    a. Infection of the testes caused by viral or bacterial infection or injury.

    b. Acute or chronic inflammation of the prostate gland

    c. Failure to initiate or maintain an erection.

    d. Enlargement of the prostate gland

31. Which of the following is a common benign tumor of the breast?

    a. Endometriosis

    b. Ectopic pregnancy

    c. Fibroadenoma

    d. Placenta previa

32. What is the primary symptom of fibroadenoma?

    a. Painful menstrual periods

    b. Absence of menstruation

    c. Enlargement of the prostate gland

    d. A benign lump in the breast

33. What is the primary symptom of amenorrhea?

    a. Painful menstrual periods

    b. Absence of menstruation

    c. Enlargement of the prostate gland

    d. A benign lump in the breast

34. What is the primary symptom of endometriosis?

    a. Painful menstrual periods

    b. Absence of menstruation

    c. Enlargement of the prostate gland

    d. A benign lump in the breast

35. What is the primary symptom of ectopic pregnancy?

    a.   Painful menstrual periods

    b.   Absence of menstruation

    c.   Painful bleeding

    d.   A benign lump in the breast

36. What is the primary symptom of miscarriage?

    a.   Painful menstrual periods

    b.   Absence of menstruation

    c.   Painful bleeding

    d.   A benign lump in the breast

37. What is the primary symptom of placenta previa?

    a.   Painful menstrual periods

    b.   Absence of menstruation

    c.   Painful bleeding

    d.   Enlargement of the uterus

38. What is the primary symptom of orchitis?

    a.   Pain and swelling of the testes.

    b.   Pain and swelling of the prostate gland.

    c.   Painful bleeding

    d.   Enlargement of the testes

39. What is the primary symptom of prostatitis?

    a.   Pain and swelling of the testes.

    b.   Pain and swelling of the prostate gland.

    c.   Painful bleeding

    d.   Enlargement of the prostate gland

40. What is the primary symptom of benign prostatic hyperplasia?

    a. Pain and swelling of the testes.

    b. Pain and swelling of the prostate gland.

    c. Urinary obstruction

    d. Enlargement of the prostate gland

41. What is the importance of professional communication with patients/clients?

    a. It helps to build trust and rapport.

    b. It helps to save time.

    c. It helps to reduce costs.

    d. It helps to increase profits.

42. Why is it important for office staff members to ask for feedback when communicating with patients?

    a. It keeps everyone engaged.

    b. It helps to clarify any misunderstandings.

    c. It helps to save time.

    d. It helps to reduce costs.

43. What is the importance of eye contact and body language in in-person communication with patients?

    a. It helps to build trust and rapport.

    b. It helps to save time.

    c. It helps to reduce costs.

    d. It helps to increase profits.

44. What is e-mail short for?

    a. Electronic mail

    b. Efficient mail

    c. Effective mail

    d. Easy mail

45. Is e-mail considered an informal type of communication?

    a. Yes

    b. No

    c. It depends on the situation.

    d. None of the above

46. What should you include in the subject line of an e-mail?

    a. The recipient's name.

    b. The sender's name.

    c. The purpose of the message

    d. The date and time

47. Is it appropriate to write an e-mail message in all upper-case letters?

    a. Yes

    b. No

    c. It depends on the situation.

    d. None of the above

48. What should you do before clicking "send" on an e-mail message?

    a. Check the recipient's name.

    b. Check the sender's name.

    c. Check the subject line.

    d. All of the above

49. What should you use in an e-mail message to show politeness?

    a. Slang words

    b. Abbreviations

    c. "Please" and "thank you."

    d. None of the above

50. Can e-mail be used as a legal document?

    a.   Yes

    b.   No

    c.   It depends on the situation.

    d.   None of the above

51. What should you avoid doing in an e-mail message?

    a.   Threatening or intimidating someone

    b.   Using humor

    c.   Using slang words

    d.   All of the above

52. What is the primary benefit of using e-mail for communication?

    a.   It is quick and easy.

    b.   It is more personal than other forms of communication.

    c.   It is more formal than other forms of communication.

    d.   It is more secure than other forms of communication.

53. What should you do if you are unsure about the appropriateness of an e-mail message?

    a.   Send it anyway.

    b.   Ask a colleague for their opinion.

    c.   Delete it and start over

    d.   None of the above

54. What is the primary disadvantage of using e-mail for communication?

    a.   It can be easily misunderstood.

    b.   It is too formal.

    c.   It is too time-consuming.

    d.   It is not secure.

55. What is the purpose of using a personal name in an e-mail message?

    a. To show politeness

    b. To make the message more personal

    c. To make the message more formal

    d. None of the above

56. What is the purpose of filling in the subject line of an e-mail message?

    a. To identify the message

    b. To show politeness

    c. To make the message more personal

    d. None of the above

57. What is the primary benefit of using body language in in-person communication?

    a. It can convey emotions and attitudes.

    b. It can save time.

    c. It can reduce costs.

    d. It can increase profits.

58. What is the primary disadvantage of using body language in in-person communication?

    a. It can be misinterpreted.

    b. It is too formal.

    c. It is too time-consuming.

    d. It is not secure.

59. What is the primary benefit of using eye contact in in-person communication?

    a. It can convey interest and attention.

    b. It can save time.

    c. It can reduce costs.

    d. It can increase profits.

60. What is the primary disadvantage of using eye contact in in-person communication?

    a. It can be misinterpreted.

    b. It is too formal.

    c. It is too time-consuming.

    d. It is not secure.

61. What is the primary benefit of asking for feedback in communication with patients?

    a. It can clarify any misunderstandings.

    b. It can save time.

    c. It can reduce costs.

    d. It can increase profits.

62. What is the primary disadvantage of asking for feedback in communication with patients?

    a. It can be time-consuming.

    b. It can be too formal.

    c. It can be too personal.

    d. None of the above

63. What is the primary benefit of using a personal name in an e-mail message?

    a. To show politeness

    b. To make the message more personal

    c. To make the message more formal

    d. None of the above

64. What is the primary disadvantage of using a personal name in an e-mail message?

    a. It can be too personal.

    b. It can be misinterpreted.

    c. It can be too formal.

    d. None of the above

65. What is the primary benefit of using "please" and "thank you" in an e-mail message?

   a. To show politeness

   b. To make the message more personal

   c. To make the message more formal

   d. None of the above

66. What is the primary disadvantage of using "please" and "thank you" in an e-mail message?

   a. It can be too personal.

   b. It can be misinterpreted.

   c. It can be too formal.

   d. None of the above

67. What is the primary benefit of using e-mail for legal purposes?

   a. It is quick and easy.

   b. It is more personal than other forms of communication.

   c. It is more formal than other forms of communication.

   d. It is more secure than other forms of communication.

68. What is the primary disadvantage of using e-mail for legal purposes?

   a. It can be easily misunderstood.

   b. It is too formal.

   c. It is too time-consuming.

   d. It is not secure.

69. What is the primary benefit of using body language in in-person communication?

   a. It can convey emotions and attitudes.

   b. It can save time.

   c. It can reduce costs.

   d. It can increase profits.

70. What is the primary disadvantage of using body language in in-person communication?

    a. It can be misinterpreted.

    b. It is too formal.

    c. It is too time-consuming.

    d. It is not secure.

71. What is the first piece of information a medical assistant should collect when scheduling a new patient?

    a. Provider and type of appointment

    b. Patient's address

    c. Reason for visit

    d. Type of insurance

72. What is the definition of fixed appointment scheduling?

    a. Scheduling a group of patients to come in at the same time.

    b. Scheduling one patient for a specific appointment time

    c. Scheduling two patients to see the same physician at once.

    d. Scheduling patients for the first half of each hour

73. What is the method of scheduling where patients are scheduled around the same block of time?

    a. Fixed appointment scheduling

    b. Cluster scheduling

    c. Double booking

    d. Wave scheduling

74. When is double booking typically used?

    a. To schedule a group of patients to come in at the same time.

    b. To schedule one patient for a specific appointment time

    c. To accommodate an emergency patient or other situations at the physician's discretion

    d. To schedule patients for the first half of each hour

75. What is the method of scheduling where patients are seen in the order they arrive?

    a. Fixed appointment scheduling

    b. Cluster scheduling

    c. Double booking

    d. Wave scheduling

76. What is the term for prioritizing patients based on their medical needs?

    a. Triage

    b. Cluster scheduling

    c. Double booking

    d. Wave scheduling

77. What is the definition of an established patient?

    a. A patient who has not received care from any healthcare providers of the same specialty within the previous 3 years.

    b. A patient who has received care from one of the healthcare providers of the same specialty in a medical office within the previous 3 years.

    c. A patient who has received major injuries due to a car accident, job-related incident, or any other accident.

    d. A patient who has never received medical care before.

78. What is the definition of a new patient?

    a. A patient who has not received care from any healthcare providers of the same specialty within the previous 3 years.

    b. A patient who has received care from one of the healthcare providers of the same specialty in a medical office within the previous 3 years.

    c. A patient who has received major injuries due to a car accident, job-related incident, or any other accident.

    d. A patient who has never received medical care before.

79. What information should a medical assistant collect when scheduling a new patient?

    a. Provider and type of appointment, correct spelling of patient's full name, patient's address, appropriate telephone number, reason for visit, name of referring physician (if available), type of insurance.

    b. Provider and type of appointment, patient's address, reason for visit, type of insurance

    c. Correct spelling of patient's full name, appropriate telephone number, name of referring physician (if available)

    d. Provider and type of appointment, correct spelling of patient's full name, patient's address, appropriate telephone number

80. What is the method of scheduling where patients are scheduled for the first half of each hour?

    a. Fixed appointment scheduling

    b. Cluster scheduling

    c. Double booking

    d. Wave scheduling

81. What is the term for a communication tool used in healthcare settings that stands for Situation, Background, Assessment, and Recommendation?

    a. SOAP

    b. HIPAA

    c. SBAR

    d. Jargon

82. What is the federal law that protects the privacy and security of patients' health information?

    a. SOAP

    b. HIPAA

    c. SBAR

    d. Jargon

83. What is the method used to document patient encounters in medical records that stands for Subjective, Objective, Assessment, and Plan?

    a. SOAP

    b. HIPAA

    c. SBAR

    d. Jargon

84. What is the term for specialized language or terminology used in a particular field, such as medical terminology?

    a. SOAP

    b. HIPAA

    c. SBAR

    d. Jargon

85. What is the term for understanding and sharing the feelings of others, and is an important skill for healthcare professionals?

    a. Empathy

    b. Sympathy

    c. Compassion

    d. Triage

86. What is the acronym for Health Insurance Portability and Accountability Act, a federal law that protects the privacy and security of patients' health information?

    a. SOAP

    b. HIPAA

    c. SBAR

    d. Jargon

87. What is the method used to document patient encounters in medical records that stands for Subjective, Objective, Assessment, and Plan?

    a. SOAP

    b. HIPAA

    c. SBAR

    d. Jargon

88. What is the term for specialized language or terminology used in a particular field, such as medical terminology?

    a. Jargon

    b. Slang

    c. Colloquialism

    d. Vernacular

89. What is the term for understanding and sharing the feelings of others, and is an important skill for healthcare professionals?

    a. Empathy

    b. Sympathy

    c. Compassion

    d. Triage

90. What is the acronym for Situation, Background, Assessment, and Recommendation, a communication tool used in healthcare settings?

    a. SOAP

    b. HIPAA

    c. SBAR

    d. Jargon

91. What is the term for the response or reaction to a message, and can be verbal or nonverbal?

    a. Feedback

    b. Noise

    c. Context

    d. Channel

92. What is the term for the method or medium used to transmit the message, such as face-to-face communication, email, or phone?

    a. Channel

    b. Feedback

    c. Context

    d. Noise

93. What is the term for any interference or distraction that can affect the communication process, such as background noise or language barriers?

    a. Noise

    b. Feedback

    c. Context

    d. Channel

94. What is the term for the situation or environment in which the communication takes place, and can include cultural, social, and physical factors?

    a.   Context

    b.   Feedback

    c.   Channel

    d.   Noise

95. What is the purpose of communication in healthcare settings?

    a.   To exchange information, build relationships, and provide care to patients.

    b.   To make small talk and pass the time.

    c.   To gossip about patients and colleagues

    d.   To avoid conflict and confrontation

96. What is the term for the ability to communicate effectively, which is a crucial skill for medical assistants as they interact with patients, physicians, and other healthcare professionals on a daily basis?

    a.   Communication skills

    b.   Technical skills

    c.   Interpersonal skills

    d.   Leadership skills

97. What is the term for paying attention to the speaker, asking clarifying questions, and providing feedback to ensure understanding?

    a.   Active listening

    b.   Passive listening

    c.   Selective listening

    d.   Inactive listening

98. What is the term for nonverbal communication, which includes body language, facial expressions, and tone of voice, and can convey emotions and attitudes?

    a.   Nonverbal communication

    b.   Verbal communication

    c.   Written communication

    d.   Visual communication

99. What is the term for verbal communication, which includes speaking and listening, and is essential for effective communication in healthcare settings?

    a. Verbal communication

    b. Nonverbal communication

    c. Written communication

    d. Visual communication

100. What is the term for the person who receives and interprets the message in the communication process?

    a. Receiver

    b. Sender

    c. Feedback

    d. Channel

PART-THREE

ANSWER TO MEDICAL ASSISTANT QUESTIONS

1. **Answer D**

    An inflammation of the genital mucous membrane of male and female - Gonorrhea is a contagious inflammation of the genital mucous membrane of male and female that must be treated to prevent further spreading of STD.

2. **Answer A**

    A serious sexually transmitted disease - Syphilis is a serious sexually transmitted disease. Infection in pregnant women can cause birth defects.

3. **Answer A**

    By direct sexual contact - HIV is transferred by direct sexual contact, by contaminated intravenous needles and syringes, or by blood transfusions that have contaminated blood.

4. **Answer B**

    A blood test - Diagnosis of HIV is by a blood test.

5. **Answer C**

    A result of the HIV virus - AIDS is ultimately a result of the HIV virus. AIDS is marked by opportunistic infections that would otherwise be eliminated by a healthy individual's immune response.

6. **Answer C**

    Inflammation and serious infection of organs in the pelvic cavity - Pelvic inflammatory disease is inflammation and serious infection of organs in the pelvic cavity. It is caused mostly in young nulliparous females and is not related to pregnancy.

7. **Answer A**

    Inflammation and infection of the vaginal tissues - Vaginitis is an inflammation and/or infection of the vaginal tissues. It is common in all ages and characterized by vaginal discharge that can be clear, greenish-yellow, and foul-smelling.

8. **Answer B**

A condition that causes cessation of menstrual periods - Menopause is the cessation of menstrual periods.

9. **Answer D**

10 years - The chronic asymptomatic or latency phase of AIDS lasts an average of 10 years.

10. **Answer D**

AIDS - The ultimate result of the HIV virus is AIDS.

11. **Answer C**

Sexual activity - The most common cause of pelvic inflammatory disease is sexual activity.

12. **Answer C**

Foul-smelling vaginal discharge - The characteristic symptom of vaginitis is foul-smelling vaginal discharge.

13. **Answer D**

Inflammation of the genital mucous membrane of male and female - The primary symptom of gonorrhea is inflammation of the genital mucous membrane of male and femal.

14. **Answer D**

Sores or rash on the genitals or mouth - The primary symptom of syphilis is sores or rash on the genitals or mouth.

15. **Answer A**

Sexual contact - The primary mode of transmission for HIV is sexual contact.

16. **Answer C**

Cessation of menstrual periods - The primary symptom of menopause is cessation of menstrual periods.

17. **Answer D**

No symptoms are present - The chronic asymptomatic or latency phase of AIDS has no symptoms present.

18. **Answer D**

Opportunistic infections that would otherwise be eliminated by a healthy individual's immune response - The primary symptom of the AIDS phase is opportunistic infections that would otherwise be eliminated by a healthy individual's immune response.

19. **Answer A**

Sexual contact - The primary mode of transmission for syphilis is sexual contact.

20. **Answer C**

Pain in the lower abdomen - The primary symptom of pelvic inflammatory disease is pain in the lower abdomen.

21. **Answer B**

A benign tumor of the breast

Fibroadenoma is a common benign tumor of the breast that is usually painless but can be painful at the time of the menstrual period.

22. **Answer B**

Absence of menstruation at puberty

Amenorrhea is the absence of the onset of menstruation at puberty or the cessation or interruption of menstruation in adulthood.

23. **Answer C**

Proliferation of endometrial tissue outside of the uterus

Endometriosis is the proliferation of endometrial tissue outside of the uterus, which can cause pain and infertility.

24. **Answer D**

Implantation of the fertilized ovum outside the uterus

Ectopic pregnancy is the implantation of the fertilized ovum outside the uterus, most commonly in the Fallopian tubes, which can be life-threatening if not treated promptly.

25. **Answer C**

Spontaneous abortion

Miscarriage is a spontaneous abortion, commonly a result of genetic abnormality.

26. Answer D

Implantation of the placenta in the lower uterine segment on the internal cervical lining

Placenta previa is the implantation of the placenta in the lower uterine segment on the internal cervical lining, which can cause painless bleeding.

27. **Answer A**

Infection of the testes caused by viral or bacterial infection or injury.

Orchitis is an infection of the testes caused by viral or bacterial infection or injury, which can cause pain and swelling.

28. **Answer B**

Acute or chronic inflammation of the prostate gland

Prostatitis is acute or chronic inflammation of the prostate gland, which can cause pain and difficulty urinating.

29. **Answer C**

Failure to initiate or maintain an erection.

Impotence is the failure to initiate or maintain an erection, which can be caused by physical or psychological factors.

30. **Answer D**

Enlargement of the prostate gland

Benign prostatic hyperplasia is the enlargement of the prostate gland, which can cause urinary obstruction and difficulty urinating.

31. **Answer C**

Fibroadenoma

Fibroadenoma is a common benign tumor of the breast.

32. **Answer D**

A benign lump in the breast

The primary symptom of fibroadenoma is a benign lump in the breast.

33. **Answer B**

Absence of menstruation

The primary symptom of amenorrhea is the absence of menstruation.

34. **Answer A**

Painful menstrual periods

The primary symptom of endometriosis is painful menstrual periods.

35. **Answer C**

Painful bleeding

The primary symptom of ectopic pregnancy is painful bleeding.

36. **Answer C**

Painful bleeding

The primary symptom of miscarriage is painful bleeding.

37. Answer C

Painful bleeding

The primary symptom of placenta previa is painless bleeding.

38. Answer A

Pain and swelling of the testes.

The primary symptom of orchitis is pain and swelling of the testes.

39. Answer B

Pain and swelling of the prostate gland.

The primary symptom of prostatitis is pain and swelling of the prostate gland.

40. Answer C

Urinary obstruction

The primary symptom of benign prostatic hyperplasia is urinary obstruction.

41. Answer A

The ability to communicate effectively is a crucial skill for medical assistants as they interact with patients, physicians, and other healthcare professionals on a daily basis.

42. Answer B

Active listening involves paying attention to the speaker, asking clarifying questions, and providing feedback to ensure understanding.

43. Answer A

Nonverbal communication includes body language, facial expressions, and tone of voice, and can convey emotions and attitudes.

44. Answer C

Written communication includes emails, letters, and other forms of written correspondence.

45. Answer B

Verbal communication includes speaking and listening and is essential for effective communication in healthcare settings.

46. Answer A

The sender is the person who initiates the communication, while the receiver is the person who receives and interprets the message.

47. Answer D

Feedback is the response or reaction to a message and can be verbal or nonverbal.

48. Answer C

The channel is the method or medium used to transmit the message, such as face-to-face communication, email, or phone.

49. Answer B

Noise refers to any interference or distraction that can affect the communication process, such as background noise or language barriers.

50. Answer A

The context refers to the situation or environment in which the communication takes place, and can include cultural, social, and physical factors.

51. Answer C

The purpose of communication in healthcare settings is to exchange information, build relationships, and provide care to patients.

52. Answer B

The tone of voice can convey emotions and attitudes and can affect the interpretation of the message.

53. Answer A

Jargon refers to specialized language or terminology used in a particular field, such as medical terminology.

54. Answer D

Empathy involves understanding and sharing the feelings of others and is an important skill for healthcare professionals.

55. Answer C

The acronym SBAR stands for Situation, Background, Assessment, and Recommendation, and is a communication tool used in healthcare settings.

56. Answer B

The acronym HIPAA stands for Health Insurance Portability and Accountability Act and is a federal law that protects the privacy and security of patients' health information.

57. Answer A

The acronym SOAP stands for Subjective, Objective, Assessment, and Plan, and is a method used to document patient encounters in medical records.

58. Answer A

Eye contact can convey interest and attention and is an important aspect of nonverbal communication.

59. Answer A

Eye contact can convey interest and attention and is an important aspect of nonverbal communication.

60. Answer A

Eye contact can be misinterpreted and may not be appropriate in all situations.

61. Answer A

Asking for feedback can clarify any misunderstandings and improve communication with patients.

62. Answer A

Asking for feedback can be time-consuming and may not be appropriate in all situations.

63. Answer B

Using a personal name in an email message can make the message more personal and build relationships.

64. Answer B

Using a personal name in an email message can be misinterpreted and may not be appropriate in all situations.

65. Answer A

Using "please" and "thank you" in an email message can show politeness and build relationships.

66. Answer A

Using "please" and "thank you" in an email message can be misinterpreted and may not be appropriate in all situations.

67. Answer D

Using email for legal purposes can be more secure than other forms of communication.

68. Answer A

Using email for legal purposes can be easily misunderstood and may not be appropriate in all situations.

69. Answer A

Body language can convey emotions and attitudes and is an important aspect of nonverbal communication.

70. Answer A

Body language can be misinterpreted and may not be appropriate in all situations.

71. Answer A.

Provider and type of appointment

72. Answer B.

Scheduling one patient for a specific appointment time

73. Answer B

Cluster scheduling

74. Answer C.

To accommodate an emergency patient or other situations at the physician's discretion

75. Answer D.

Wave scheduling

76. Answer A.

Triage

77. Answer B.

A patient who has received care from one of the healthcare providers of the same specialty in a medical office within the previous 3 years.

78. Answer A.

A patient who has not received care from any healthcare providers of the same specialty within the previous 3 years.

79. Answer A.

Provider and type of appointment, correct spelling of patient's full name, patient's address, appropriate telephone number, reason for visit, name of referring physician (if available), type of insurance.

80. Answer D.

Wave scheduling

81. Answer C.

SBAR

82. Answer B.

HIPAA

83. Answer A.

SOAP

84. Answer D.

Jargon

85. Answer A.

Empathy

86. Answer B.

HIPAA

87. Answer A.

SOAP

88. Answer A.

Jargon

89. Answer A.

Empathy

90. Answer C.

SBAR

91. Answer A.

Feedback

92. Answer A.

Channel

93. Answer A.

Noise

94. Answer A

Context

95. Answer A

To exchange information, build relationships, and provide care to patients.

96. Answer A

Communication skills

97. Answer A

Active listening

98. Answer A

Nonverbal communication

99. Answer A

Verbal communication

100. Answer A

Receiver

MEDICAL ASSISTANT CERTIFICATION EXAMINATION STUDY GUIDE PART-FOUR

1. What type of joint is a hinge joint?

    a. Fibrous joint

    b. Cartilaginous joint

    c. Synovial joint

    d. Suture joint

2. What are bursae?

    a. Bones in a joint

    b. Muscles that move a joint

    c. Sacs of fluid were located between bones and tendons.

    d. Ligaments that hold a joint together

3. What is extension?

    a. Movement away from the midline

    b. Movement towards the midline

    c. Decrease in the angle of a joint

    d. Increase in the angle of a joint

4. What is flexion?

    a. Movement away from the midline

    b. Movement towards the midline

    c. Decrease in the angle of a joint

    d. Increase in the angle of a joint

5. What is abduction?

    a. Movement away from the midline

    b. Movement towards the midline

    c. Decrease in the angle of a joint

    d. Increase in the angle of a joint

6. What is addiction?

    a. Movement away from the midline

    b. Movement towards the midline

    c. Decrease in the angle of a joint

    d. Increase in the angle of a joint

7. What is supination?

    a. Turning the palm or foot upward

    b. Turning the palm or foot downward

    c. Raising the foot, pulling the toes toward the shin

    d. None of the above

8. What is pronation?

    a. Turning the palm or foot upward

    b. Turning the palm or foot downward

    c. Raising the foot, pulling the toes toward the shin

    d. None of the above

9. What is dorsiflexion?

    a. Turning the palm or foot upward

    b. Turning the palm or foot downward

    c. Raising the foot, pulling the toes toward the shin

    d. None of the above

10. What is the normal anatomic position?

    a. Lying on the back

    b. Lying on the stomach

    c. Standing with arms lank and palms forward

    d. Sitting with feet supported on a footrest or stool.

11. What is the sitting position?

    a. Lying on the back

    b. Lying on the stomach

    c. Standing with arms lank and palms forward

    d. Sitting with feet supported on a footrest or stool.

12. What is the supine position?

    a. Lying on the back

    b. Lying on the stomach

    c. Standing with arms lank and palms forward

    d. Sitting with feet supported on a footrest or stool.

13. What is the prone position?

    a.   Lying on the back

    b.   Lying on the stomach

    c.   Standing with arms lank and palms forward

    d.   Sitting with feet supported on a footrest or stool.

14. What is the lateral recumbent position?

    a.   Lying on the back

    b.   Lying on the stomach

    c.   Lying on the side

    d.   Sitting with feet supported on a footrest or stool.

15. What is the dorsal recumbent position?

    a.   Lying on the back with legs separated, knees bent, and feet flat on the table.

    b.   Lying on the stomach

    c.   Standing with arms lank and palms forward

    d.   Sitting with feet supported on a footrest or stool.

16. What is the lithotomy position?

    a.   Lying on the back with legs separated, knees bent, and feet flat on the table.

    b.   Lying on the stomach

    c.   Lying on the left side with the left arm and shoulder in a prone position

    d.   Half-sitting with the head of an examination table elevated at 90 degrees.

17. What is the Sim's position?

    a.   Lying on the back with legs separated, knees bent, and feet flat on the table.

    b.   Lying on the stomach

    c.   Lying on the left side with the left arm and shoulder in a prone position

    d.   Half-sitting with the head of an examination table elevated at 90 degrees.

18. What is the Fowler position?

    a.   Lying on the back with legs separated, knees bent, and feet flat on the table.

    b.   Lying on the stomach

    c.   Lying on the left side with the left arm and shoulder in a prone position

    d.   Half-sitting with the head of an examination table elevated at 90 degrees.

19. Which type of joint is surrounded by joint capsules?

    a.   Fibrous joint

    b.   Cartilaginous joint

    c.   Synovial joint

    d.   Suture joint

20. What is the purpose of bursae?

    a.   To hold a joint together

    b.   To move a joint

    c.   To provide cushioning between bones and tendons

    d.   None of the above

21. What is the opposite of extension?

   a. Flexion

   b. Abduction

   c. Adduction

   d. Supination

22. What is the opposite of abduction?

   a. Flexion

   b. Extension

   c. Adduction

   d. Pronation

23. What is the opposite of supination?

   a. Pronation

   b. Dorsiflexion

   c. Extension

   d. Abduction

24. What is the opposite of dorsiflexion?

   a. Plantarflexion

   b. Extension

   c. Adduction

   d. Abduction

25. Which body position involves lying on the stomach?

    a. Supine position

    b. Prone position

    c. Lateral recumbent position

    d. Dorsal recumbent position

26. Which body position involves lying on the side?

    a. Supine position

    b. Prone position

    c. Lateral recumbent position

    d. Dorsal recumbent position

27. Which body position involves lying on the back with legs separated, knees bent, and feet flat on the table?

    a. Supine position

    b. Prone position

    c. Lateral recumbent position

    d. Dorsal recumbent position

28. Which body position involves lying on the left side with the left arm and shoulder in a prone position?

    a. Supine position

    b. Prone position

    c. Lateral recumbent position

    d. Sim's position

29. Which body position involves half-sitting with the head of an examination table elevated at 90 degrees?

   a. Fowler position

   b. Lithotomy position

   c. Sim's position

   d. Dorsal recumbent position

30. Which type of joint is commonly found in the knee?

   a. Fibrous joint

   b. Cartilaginous joint

   c. Synovial joint

   d. Suture

31. What is the normal anatomic position?

   a. Standing with arms lank and palms forward

   b. Lying on the back

   c. Sitting with feet supported on a footrest or stool.

   d. Lying on the stomach

32. What is the supine position?

   a. Lying on the back

   b. Lying on the stomach

   c. Lying on the side

   d. Half-sitting with the head of an examination table elevated at 90 degrees.

33. What is the prone position?

    a.   Lying on the stomach

    b.   Lying on the back

    c.   Lying on the side

    d.   Half-sitting with the head of an examination table elevated at 90 degrees.

34. What is the lateral recumbent position?

    a.   Lying on the back

    b.   Lying on the stomach

    c.   Lying on the side

    d.   Half-sitting with the head of an examination table elevated at 90 degrees.

35. What is the dorsal recumbent position?

    a.   Lying on the back with legs separated, knees bent, and feet flat on the table.

    b.   Lying on the stomach

    c.   Lying on the side

    d.   Half-sitting with the head of an examination table elevated at 90 degrees.

36. What is the lithotomy position?

    a.   Lying on the back

    b.   Lying on the stomach

    c.   Lying on the side

    d.   Lying on the back with legs separated, knees bent, and feet flat on the table, but patient's feet are in stirrups.

37. What is the Sim's position?

    a. Lying on the back

    b. Lying on the stomach

    c. Lying on the side

    d. Half-sitting with the head of an examination table elevated at 90 degrees.

38. What is the Fowler position?

    a. Lying on the back

    b. Lying on the stomach

    c. Lying on the side

    d. Half-sitting with the head of an examination table elevated at 90 degrees.

39. What is a synovial joint?

    a. A joint that allows movement in only one plane

    b. A joint that is surrounded by joint capsules that contain synovial fluid.

    c. A joint that allows movement in multiple planes

    d. A joint that is immovable

40. What are bursae?

    a. Small fluid-filled sacs that reduce friction between bones and tendons or muscles around a joint

    b. Small fluid-filled sacs that provide cushioning between bones and tendons or muscles around a joint

    c. Small fluid-filled sacs that contain synovial fluid.

    d. Small fluid-filled sacs that are immovable.

41. What is extension?

       a.   Movement away from the midline

       b.   Movement towards the midline

       c.   Increase in the angle of a joint

       d.   Decrease in the angle of a joint

42. What is flexion?

       a.   Movement away from the midline

       b.   Movement towards the midline

       c.   Decrease in the angle of a joint

       d.   Increase in the angle of a joint

43. What is abduction?

       a.   Movement away from the midline

       b.   Movement towards the midline

       c.   Increase in the angle of a joint

       d.   Decrease in the angle of a joint

44. What is adduction?

       a.   Movement towards the midline

       b.   Movement away from the midline

       c.   Increase in the angle of a joint

       d.   Decrease in the angle of a joint

45. What is rotation?

    a.   Movement towards the midline

    b.   Movement away from the midline

    c.   Circular movement around an axis

    d.   Increase in the angle of a joint

46. What is circumduction?

    a.   Movement towards the midline

    b.   Movement away from the midline

    c.   Circular movement around an axis

    d.   Increase in the angle of a joint

47. What is the purpose of range of motion exercises?

    a.   To increase muscle strength

    b.   To increase joint flexibility

    c.   To decrease joint pain

    d.   All of the above

48. What is the purpose of passive range of motion exercises?

    a.   To increase muscle strength

    b.   To increase joint flexibility

    c.   To decrease joint pain

    d.   To improve coordination

49. What is the purpose of active range of motion exercises?

   a. To increase muscle strength

   b. To increase joint flexibility

   c. To decrease joint pain

   d. To improve coordination

50. What is the purpose of resistive range of motion exercises?

   a. To increase muscle strength

   b. To increase joint flexibility

   c. To decrease joint pain

   d. To improve coordination

51. What is the purpose of isometric exercises?

   a. To increase muscle strength

   b. To increase joint flexibility

   c. To decrease joint pain

   d. To improve coordination

52. What is the purpose of isotonic exercises?

   a. To increase muscle strength

   b. To increase joint flexibility

   c. To decrease joint pain

   d. To improve coordination

53. What is the purpose of isokinetic exercises?

   a. To increase muscle strength

   b. To increase joint flexibility

   c. To decrease joint pain

   d. To improve coordination

54. What is the purpose of stretching exercises?

   a. To increase muscle strength

   b. To increase joint flexibility

   c. To decrease joint pain

   d. To improve coordination

55. What is the purpose of aerobic exercises?

   a. To increase muscle strength

   b. To increase joint flexibility

   c. To improve cardiovascular endurance

   d. To improve coordination

56. What is the purpose of anaerobic exercises?

   a. To increase muscle strength

   b. To increase joint flexibility

   c. To improve cardiovascular endurance

   d. To improve coordination

57. What is the purpose of balance exercises?

    a. To increase muscle strength

    b. To increase joint flexibility

    c. To improve balance and stability

    d. To improve coordination

58. What is the purpose of coordination exercises?

    a. To increase muscle strength

    b. To increase joint flexibility

    c. To improve balance and stability

    d. To improve coordination

59. What is the purpose of proprioceptive exercises?

    a. To increase muscle strength

    b. To increase joint flexibility

    c. To improve balance and stability

    d. To improve proprioception

60. What is the purpose of resistance training?

    a. To increase muscle strength

    b. To increase joint flexibility

    c. To improve balance and stability

    d. To improve cardiovascular endurance

61. What is the purpose of a sliding glass window in a medical office?

    a. To prevent patients from seeing the receptionist

    b. To prevent patients from hearing conversations in the reception area

    c. To provide a clear view of the waiting room

    d. To allow for better ventilation in the office

62. Why should only one patient be at the front desk or window at a time?

    a. To prevent patients from overhearing conversations

    b. To make the receptionist's job easier

    c. To reduce the risk of patient confusion

    d. To allow for better communication between patients

63. What should a medical assistant do if it is necessary to discuss sensitive information with a patient?

    a. Speak quietly at the front desk.

    b. Take the patient to a private area.

    c. Ask the patient to come back later.

    d. Discuss the information over the phone.

64. What is the purpose of authentication in computer network security?

    a. To allow users to access any part of the network.

    b. To prevent unauthorized access to the network

    c. To make it easier for users to remember their passwords.

    d. To allow users to share their passwords with others.

65. What are the levels of authorization in computer network security?

    a. Different types of passwords

    b. Different levels of access to the network

    c. Different types of computer hardware

    d. Different types of software programs

66. Why is it important for medical offices to provide secure access to patient information?

    a. To protect patient privacy

    b. To make it easier for medical assistants to access information.

    c. To reduce the risk of computer viruses

    d. To improve the speed of the computer network

67. What is the purpose of a password in computer network security?

    a. To allow users to access any part of the network.

    b. To prevent unauthorized access to the network

    c. To make it easier for users to remember their usernames.

    d. To allow users to share their passwords with others.

68. What should a medical assistant do if a patient asks for information about another patient?

    a. Provide information if it is not sensitive.

    b. Refuse to provide the information.

    c. Ask the patient to come back later.

    d. Discuss the information over the phone.

69. What is the purpose of a separate room for scheduling appointments?

   a. To provide a quiet space for patients

   b. To prevent patients from hearing conversations in the reception area

   c. To allow for better communication between patients

   d. To provide a clear view of the waiting room

70. What should a medical assistant do if a patient overhears a conversation at the front desk?

   a. Apologize and explain the situation.

   b. Ignore the patient and continue the conversation.

   c. Ask the patient to leave the office.

   d. Discuss the information over the phone.

71. What is the purpose of HIPAA regulations?

   a. To protect patient privacy

   b. To make it easier for medical assistants to access information.

   c. To reduce the risk of computer viruses

   d. To improve the speed of the computer network

72. What should a medical assistant do if a patient asks for their own medical records?

   a. Provide the records immediately.

   b. Refuse to provide the records.

   c. Ask the patient to come back later.

   d. Discuss the records over the phone.

73. What is the purpose of secure access to patient information?

    a. To protect patient privacy

    b. To make it easier for medical assistants to access information.

    c. To reduce the risk of computer viruses

    d. To improve the speed of the computer network

74. What should a medical assistant do if they accidentally disclose patient information to the wrong person?

    a. Apologize and explain the situation.

    b. Ignore the mistake and continue working.

    c. Ask the patient to come back later.

    d. Discuss the information over the phone.

75. What is the purpose of a log in for computer network security?

    a. To allow users to access any part of the network.

    b. To prevent unauthorized access to the network

    c. To make it easier for users to remember their passwords.

    d. To allow users to share their passwords with others.

76. What should a medical assistant do if they receive a phone call from someone asking for patient information?

    a. Provide information if it is not sensitive.

    b. Refuse to provide the information.

    c. Ask the caller to come to the office in person.

    d. Discuss the information over the phone.

77. What is the purpose of a private area for discussing sensitive information?

    a. To protect patient privacy

    b. To make it easier for medical assistants to communicate

    c. To reduce the risk of computer viruses

    d. To improve the speed of the computer network

78. What should a medical assistant do if they suspect a breach of patient confidentiality?

    a. Report the incident to their supervisor.

    b. Ignore the situation and continue working.

    c. Ask the patient to come back later.

    d. Discuss the information over the phone.

79. What is the purpose of a secure computer network in a medical office?

    a. To protect patient privacy

    b. To make it easier for medical assistants to access information.

    c. To reduce the risk of computer viruses

    d. To improve the speed of the computer network

80. What should a medical assistant do if they receive an email requesting patient information?

    a. Provide information if it is not sensitive.

    b. Refuse to provide the information.

    c. Ask the sender to come to the office in person.

    d. Discuss the information over email.

81. What is the documentation method where physicians write notes on the patient encounter and then have those notes added to a patient's medical record?

   a. SOAP note charting

   b. POMR charting

   c. Narrative style charting

   d. None of the above

82. What does SOAP stand for in SOAP note charting?

   a. Subjective, objective, assessment, plan

   b. Symptoms, observations, assessment, plan

   c. Subjective, objective, analysis, plan

   d. Symptoms, observations, analysis, plan

83. Which type of information is considered subjective in SOAP note charting?

   a. Information based on observations made by the physician or medical assistant.

   b. Laboratory results or vital signs

   c. A summary of the patient's symptoms

   d. None of the above

84. Which type of information is considered objective in SOAP note charting?

   a. Information based on observations made by the physician or medical assistant.

   b. Laboratory results or vital signs

   c. A summary of the patient's symptoms

   d. None of the above

85. What is an assessment in SOAP note charting?

    a.   A summary of the patient's symptoms may often include a diagnosis as well as a list of other potential diagnoses, usually in order of most likely to least likely.

    b.   Information based on observations made by the physician or medical assistant.

    c.   A plan of action for a patient, such as prescriptions, instructions, or referrals

    d.   None of the above

86. What is a plan in SOAP note charting?

    a.   A plan of action for a patient, such as prescriptions, instructions, or referrals

    b.   Information based on observations made by the physician or medical assistant.

    c.   A summary of the patient's symptoms may often include a diagnosis as well as a list of other potential diagnoses, usually in order of most likely to least likely.

    d.   None of the above

87. What is problem-oriented medical record charting?

    a.   A method of tracking the patient's medical history and current health status

    b.   A method of adding information to a patient's medical record

    c.   A method of documenting a patient encounter using SOAP notes

    d.   None of the above

88. Which documentation method is known as the narrative style?

    a.   SOAP note charting

    b.   POMR charting

    c.   Problem-oriented medical record charting

    d.   None of the above

89. Which type of information is considered objective in narrative style charting?

    a. Information based on observations made by the physician or medical assistant.

    b. Laboratory results or vital signs

    c. A summary of the patient's symptoms

    d. None of the above

90. Which type of information is considered subjective in narrative style charting?

    a. Information based on observations made by the physician or medical assistant.

    b. Laboratory results or vital signs

    c. A summary of the patient's symptoms

    d. None of the above

91. Which documentation method is known as SOAP note charting?

    a. Narrative style charting

    b. POMR charting

    c. Problem-oriented medical record charting

    d. None of the above

92. What does POMR stand for?

    a. Problem-oriented medical record charting

    b. Patient-oriented medical record charting

    c. Physician-oriented medical record charting

    d. None of the above

93. Which type of information is considered subjective in POMR charting?

    a. Information based on observations made by the physician or medical assistant.

    b. Laboratory results or vital signs

    c. A summary of the patient's symptoms

    d. None of the above

94. Which type of information is considered objective in POMR charting?

    a. Information based on observations made by the physician or medical assistant.

    b. Laboratory results or vital signs

    c. A summary of the patient's symptoms

    d. None of the above

95. What is an assessment in POMR charting?

    a. A summary of the patient's symptoms may often include a diagnosis as well as a list of other potential diagnoses, usually in order of most likely to least likely.

    b. Information based on observations made by the physician or medical assistant.

    c. A plan of action for a patient, such as prescriptions, instructions, or referrals

    d. None of the above

96. What is a plan in POMR charting?

    a. A plan of action for a patient, such as prescriptions, instructions, or referrals

    b. Information based on observations made by the physician or medical assistant.

    c. A summary of the patient's symptoms may often include a diagnosis as well as a list of other potential diagnoses, usually in order of most likely to least likely.

    d. None of the above

97. Why is documentation important in-patient care?

    a. It provides a record of the patient's medical history and current health status.

    b. It helps healthcare providers make informed decisions about patient care.

    c. It helps ensure continuity of care between healthcare providers.

    d. All of the above

98. What is the purpose of SOAP note charting?

    a. To provide a structured method of documenting a patient encounter

    b. To provide a narrative of the patient encounter

    c. To track the patient's medical history and current health status

    d. None of the above

99. What is the purpose of POMR charting?

    a. To provide a structured method of documenting a patient encounter

    b. To provide a narrative of the patient encounter

    c. To track the patient's medical history and current health status

    d. None of the above

100.Which type of information is considered most important in SOAP note charting?

    a. Subjective information

    b. Objective information

    c. Assessment information

    d. Plan information

PART-FOUR

ANSWER TO MEDICAL ASSISTANT QUESTIONS

1. Answer: C

    Synovial joint - A hinge joint is a type of synovial joint that allows movement in only one plane, like a door hinge.

2. Answer: C

    Sacs of fluid located between bones and tendons - Bursae are small fluid-filled sacs that reduce friction between bones and tendons or muscles around a joint.

3. Answer: D

    Increase in the angle of a joint - Extension is the movement that increases the angle between two bones at a joint.

4. Answer: C

    Decrease in the angle of a joint - Flexion is the movement that decreases the angle between two bones at a joint.

5. Answer: A

    Movement away from the midline - Abduction is the movement of a body part away from the midline of the body.

6. Answer: B

    Movement towards the midline - Adduction is the movement of a body part towards the midline of the body.

7. Answer: A

    Turning the palm or foot upward - Supination is the movement of the forearm or foot so that the palm or sole faces upward.

8. Answer: B

Turning the palm or foot downward - Pronation is the movement of the forearm or foot so that the palm or sole faces downward.

9. Answer: C.

Raising the foot, pulling the toes toward the shin - Dorsiflexion is the movement of the foot upwards towards the shin.

10. Answer: C

Standing with arms lank and palms forward - The normal anatomic position is the standard reference position for the body, with the arms at the sides and palms facing forward.

11. Answer: D

Sitting with feet supported on a footrest or stool - The sitting position is a seated posture with the feet supported on a footrest or stool.

12. Answer: A

Lying on the back - The supine position is a lying position with the face up and the back on a flat surface.

13. Answer: B

Lying on the stomach - The prone position is a lying position with the face down and the front of the body on a flat surface.

14. Answer: C

Lying on the side - The lateral recumbent position is a lying position on one side of the body.

15. Answer: A

Lying on the back with legs separated, knees bent, and feet flat on the table - The dorsal recumbent position is a lying position on the back with the legs separated, knees bent, and feet flat on the table.

16. Answer: A

Lying on the back with legs separated, knees bent, and feet flat on the table, but patient's feet are in stirrups - The lithotomy position is a variation of the dorsal recumbent position with the patient's feet in stirrups.

17. Answer: C

Lying on the left side with the left arm and shoulder in a prone position - The Sim's position is a lying position on the left side with the left arm and shoulder in a prone position.

18. Answer: D

. Half-sitting with head of an examination table elevated at 90 degrees - The Fowler position is a sitting position with the head of the examination table elevated at 90 degrees.

19. Answer: C

Synovial joint - Synovial joints are surrounded by joint capsules that contain synovial fluid, which lubricates the joint and reduces friction.

20. Answer: C

To provide cushioning between bones and tendons - Bursae are small fluid-filled sacs that provide cushioning between bones and tendons or muscles around a joint.

21. Answer: A

Flexion - Flexion is the movement that decreases the angle between two bones at a joint, the opposite of extension.

22. Answer: C

Adduction - Adduction is the movement of a body part towards the midline of the body, the opposite of abduction.

23. Answer: A

Pronation - Pronation is the movement of the forearm or foot so that the palm or sole faces downward, the opposite of supination.

24. Answer: A

Plantarflexion - Plantarflexion is the movement of the foot downwards away from the shin, the opposite of dorsiflexion.

25. Answer: B

Prone position - The prone position is a laying position with the face down and the front of the body on a flat surface.

26. Answer: C

Lateral recumbent position - The lateral recumbent position is a lying position on one side of the body.

27. Answer: D

Dorsal recumbent position - The dorsal recumbent position is a lying position on the back with the legs separated, knees bent, and feet flat on the table.

28. Answer: D

Sim's position - The Sim's position is a lying position on the left side with the left arm and shoulder in a prone position.

29. Answer: A

Fowler position - The Fowler position is a sitting position with the head of the examination table elevated at 90 degrees.

30. Answer: C

Synovial joint - The knee joint is a type of synovial joint that allows movement in multiple planes, including flexion, extension, and rotation.

31. Answer: A

Standing with arms lank and palms forward

32. Answer: A

Lying on the back

33. Answer: A

Lying on the stomach

34. Answer: C

Lying on the side

35. Answer: A

Lying on the back with legs separated, knees bent, and feet flat on the table.

36. Answer: D

Lying on the back with legs separated, knees bent, and feet flat on the table, but patient's feet are in stirrups.

37. Answer: C

Lying on the side with the left arm and shoulder in a prone position

38. Answer: D

Half-sitting with the head of an examination table elevated at 90 degrees.

39. Answer: B

A joint that is surrounded by joint capsules that contain synovial fluid.

40. Answer: A

Small fluid-filled sacs that reduce friction between bones and tendons or muscles around a joint

41. Answer: C.

Increase in the angle of a joint

42. Answer: C

Decrease in the angle of a joint

43. Answer: A

Movement away from the midline

44. Answer: A

   Movement towards the midline

45. Answer: C.

   Circular movement around an axis

46. Answer: C

   Circular movement around an axis

47. Answer: D

   All of the above

48. Answer: B

   To increase joint flexibility

49. Answer: A.

   To increase muscle strength

50. Answer: A

   To increase muscle strength

51. Answer: A

   To increase muscle strength

52. Answer: A

   To increase muscle strength

53. Answer: A

   To increase muscle strength

54. Answer: B

   To increase joint flexibility

55. Answer: C

   To improve cardiovascular endurance

56. Answer: A

   To increase muscle strength

57. Answer: C

   To improve balance and stability

58. Answer: D

   To improve coordination

59. Answer: D

   To improve proprioception

60. Answer: A

   To increase muscle strength

61. Answer B

   The purpose of a sliding glass window is to prevent patients from hearing conversations in the reception area.

62. Answer A

   Only one patient should be at the front desk or window at a time to prevent patients from overhearing conversations.

63. Answer B

   If it is necessary to discuss sensitive information, the patient should be taken to a private area.

64. answer B

   Authentication is used to prevent unauthorized access to the network.

65. Answer B

   Levels of authorization are used to provide different levels of access to the network.

66. Answer A

Secure access to patient information is important to protect patient privacy.

67. Answer B

A password is used to prevent unauthorized access to the network.

68. Answer B

A medical assistant should refuse to provide information about another patient to protect patient privacy.

69. Answer B

A separate room for scheduling appointments is used to prevent patients from hearing conversations in the reception area.

70. Answer A

If a patient overhears a conversation at the front desk, the medical assistant should apologize and explain the situation.

71. Answer A

HIPAA regulations are in place to protect patient privacy.

72. Answer A

A medical assistant should provide a patient's medical records immediately if requested.

73. Answer A

Secure access to patient information is important to protect patient privacy.

74. Answer A

If a medical assistant accidentally discloses patient information to the wrong person, they should apologize and explain the situation.

75. Answer B

A log in is used to prevent unauthorized access to the network.

76. Answer B

A medical assistant should refuse to provide patient information over the phone to protect patient privacy.

77. Answer A

A private area is used to protect patient privacy when discussing sensitive information. (A)

78. Answer A

If a medical assistant suspects a breach of patient confidentiality, they should report the incident to their supervisor.

79. Answer A

A secure computer network is important to protect patient privacy.

80. Answer B

A medical assistant should refuse to provide patient information over email to protect patient privacy.

81. Answer C

The documentation method where physicians write notes on the patient encounter and then have those notes added to a patient's medical record is known as the narrative style.

82. Answer A

SOAP stands for subjective, objective, assessment, and plan in SOAP note charting.

83. Answer C

Any information that the patient provides, including a chief complaint, or comments made during an examination are considered subjective information in SOAP note charting.

84. Answer A

Information based on observations made by the physician or medical assistant are considered objective in SOAP note charting.

85. Answer A

An assessment is a summary of the patient's symptoms and may often include a diagnosis as well as a list of other potential diagnoses, usually in order of most likely to least likely in SOAP note charting.

86. Answer A

A plan consists of any information regarding the prescribed plan of action for a patient, such as prescriptions, instructions, or referrals in SOAP note charting.

87. Answer B

Problem-oriented medical record charting is a method of adding information to a patient's medical record.

88. Answer C

The documentation method where physicians write notes on the patient encounter and then have those notes added to a patient's medical record is known as the narrative style.

89. Answer A

Information based on observations made by the physician or medical assistant are considered objective in narrative style charting.

90. Answer D

None of the above. There is no subjective information in narrative style charting.

91. Answer A

SOAP note charting is a documentation method where physicians write notes on the patient encounter and then have those notes added to a patient's medical record.

92. Answer A

POMR stands for problem-oriented medical record charting.

93. Answer C

A summary of the patient's symptoms is considered subjective information in POMR charting.

94. Answer A

Information based on observations made by the physician or medical assistant are considered objective in POMR charting.

95. Answer A

An assessment is a summary of the patient's symptoms and may often include a diagnosis as well as a list of other potential diagnoses, usually in order of most likely to least likely in POMR charting.

96. Answer A

A plan consists of any information regarding the prescribed plan of action for a patient, such as prescriptions, instructions, or referrals in POMR charting.

97. Answer D

Documentation is important in-patient care because it provides a record of the patient's medical history and current health status, helps healthcare providers make informed decisions about patient care, and helps ensure continuity of care between healthcare providers.

98. Answer A

- The purpose of SOAP note charting is to provide a structured method of documenting a patient encounter.

99. Answer C

The purpose of POMR charting is to track the patient's medical history and current health status.

100. Answer C

Assessment information is considered most important in SOAP note charting as it provides a summary of the patient's symptoms and may often include a diagnosis as well as a list of other potential diagnoses, usually in order of most likely to least likely.

MEDICAL ASSISTANT CERTIFICATION
EXAMINATION STUDY GUIDE
PART-FIVE

1. What is the normal range for adult respiration rate?

    a. 10-15 per minute

    b. 20-25 per minute

    c. 12-20 per minute

    d. 30-35 per minute

2. How is respiration rate measured?

    a. By counting the number of respirations per minute

    b. By measuring the amount of force exerted by the blood on the peripheral arterial walls

    c. By measuring the amount of oxygen in the blood

    d. By measuring the amount of carbon dioxide in the blood

3. What is apnea?

    a. A decrease in number of respirations

    b. A respiration rate of greater than 40/min

    c. A temporary complete absence of breathing

    d. An increase in the amount of force exerted by the blood on the peripheral arterial walls.

4. What is tachypnea?

    a. A decrease in number of respirations

    b. A respiration rate of greater than 40/min

    c. A temporary complete absence of breathing

    d. An increase in the amount of force exerted by the blood on the peripheral arterial walls.

5. What is bradypnea?

   a. A decrease in number of respirations

   b. A respiration rate of greater than 40/min

   c. A temporary complete absence of breathing

   d. An increase in the amount of force exerted by the blood on the peripheral arterial walls.

6. What is blood pressure?

   a. The measurement of the amount of force exerted by the blood on the peripheral arterial walls.

   b. The measurement of the amount of oxygen in the blood

   c. The measurement of the amount of carbon dioxide in the blood

   d. The measurement of the number of heart beats per minute

7. What are the two components of blood pressure measurement?

   a. Systole and diastole

   b. Oxygen and carbon dioxide

   c. Heartbeats and respiration rate

   d. Rate and rhythm

8. What is the normal range for adult blood pressure?

   a. 120/80 mmHg

   b. 140/90 mmHg

   c. 90/60 mmHg

   d. 160/100 mmHg

9. What is the physician listening to when checking the chest/heartbeats?

   a. Signs of abnormality in beats

   b. Signs of abnormality in respiration rate

   c. Signs of abnormality in blood pressure

   d. Signs of abnormality in oxygen levels

10. What is a murmur?

   a. An indication of valvular heart disease

   b. A decrease in number of heartbeats

   c. A temporary complete absence of breathing

   d. A respiration rate of greater than 40/min

11. What is the formula for calculating respiration rate?

   a. Count the number of respirations per minute.

   b. Multiply the number of respirations by two.

   c. Count the number of respirations for 30 seconds and multiply by two.

   d. Count the number of respirations for 1 minute.

12. What is the cause of apnea?

   a. A reduction in the stimuli to the respiratory centers of the brain

   b. A decrease in number of respirations

   c. A respiration rate of greater than 40/min

   d. An increase in the amount of force exerted by the blood on the peripheral arterial walls.

13. What is the cause of tachypnea in newborns?

    a. Hysteria

    b. Valvular heart disease

    c. Respiratory disease

    d. None of the above

14. What is the cause of bradypnea?

    a. Decrease in number of respirations during sleep.

    b. Increase in number of respirations during sleep.

    c. Respiratory disease

    d. None of the above

15. What is the unit of measurement for blood pressure?

    a. Millimeters of mercury (mmHg)

    b. Liters per minute (L/min)

    c. Beats per minute (bpm)

    d. None of the above

16. What is the purpose of measuring blood pressure?

    a. To measure the amount of oxygen in the blood

    b. To measure the amount of carbon dioxide in the blood

    c. To measure the amount of force exerted by the blood on the peripheral arterial walls.

    d. To measure the number of heart beats per minute

17. What is the difference between systolic and diastolic blood pressure?

    a.   Systolic is the highest amount of pressure exerted during the cardiac cycle, while diastolic is the lowest amount of pressure.

    b.   Systolic is the lowest amount of pressure exerted during the cardiac cycle, while diastolic is the highest amount of pressure.

    c.   Systolic and diastolic are the same thing.

    d.   None of the above.

18. What is the normal range for newborn respiration rate?

    a.   12-20 per minute

    b.   20-25 per minute

    c.   30-35 per minute

    d.   None of the above

19. What is the cause of tachypnea in adults?

    a.   Hysteria

    b.   Valvular heart disease

    c.   Respiratory disease

    d.   None of the above

20. What is the cause of apnea in adults?

    a.   A reduction in the stimuli to the respiratory centers of the brain

    b.   A decrease in number of respirations

    c.   A respiration rate of greater than 40/min

    d.   An increase in the amount of force exerted by the blood on the peripheral arterial walls.

21. Which route of medication administration involves placing medication between the cheek and gum until it dissolves?

    a.   Intradermal

    b.   Sublingual

    c.   Intramuscular

    d.   Topical

22. Which route of medication administration involves injecting medication into the muscle?

    a.   Intradermal

    b.   Subcutaneous

    c.   Intramuscular

    d.   Topical

23. Which route of medication administration involves rubbing, patting, spraying, or swabbing medication onto the skin?

    a.   Intradermal

    b.   Subcutaneous

    c.   Topical

    d.   Inhalation

24. Which route of medication administration involves instilling medication into the eyes?

    a.   Ophthalmic

    b.   Rectal

    c.   Otic

    d.   Vaginal

25. Which route of medication administration involves inserting a suppository into the rectum?

    a. Ophthalmic

    b. Rectal

    c. Otic

    d. Vaginal

26. Which route of medication administration involves administering medication as a douche?

    a. Ophthalmic

    b. Rectal

    c. Otic

    d. Vaginal

27. Which route of medication administration involves injecting medication into the subcutaneous layer of the skin at a 45-degree angle?

    a. Intradermal

    b. Subcutaneous

    c. Intramuscular

    d. Topical

28. Which route of medication administration involves inhaling medication to achieve local effects within the respiratory tract?

    a. Inhalation

    b. Ophthalmic

    c. Rectal

    d. Vaginal

29. Which route of medication administration involves injecting medication between the upper layers of the skin at a 15-degree angle?

    a. Intradermal

    b. Subcutaneous

    c. Intramuscular

    d. Topical

30. Which route of medication administration involves instilling medication (usually drops) into the ear?

    a. Ophthalmic

    b. Rectal

    c. Otic

    d. Vaginal

31. Which route of medication administration involves administering medication in the patch form for continuous absorption and effects that last over many hours?

    a. Buccal

    b. Sublingual

    c. Transdermal

    d. Inhalation

32. Which route of medication administration involves injecting medication into the muscle at a 90-degree angle and aspirating?

    a. Intradermal

    b. Subcutaneous

    c. Intramuscular

    d. Topical

33. Which route of medication administration involves administering medication as a solution into the rectum?

    a. Ophthalmic

    b. Rectal

    c. Otic

    d. Vaginal

34. Which route of medication administration involves asking the patient to place medication between their cheek and gum until it dissolves?

    a. Intradermal

    b. Sublingual

    c. Intramuscular

    d. Topical

35. Which route of medication administration involves administering medication as a solution into the vagina?

    a. Ophthalmic

    b. Rectal

    c. Otic

    d. Vaginal:

36. Which route of medication administration involves administering medication as an enema?

    a. Buccal

    b. Sublingual

    c. Transdermal

    d. Rectal

37. Which route of medication administration involves administering medication as a spray or mist into the nose?

    a. Inhalation

    b. Ophthalmic

    c. Otic

    d. Vaginal

38. Which route of medication administration involves administering medication as a solution into the urethra?

    a. Ophthalmic

    b. Rectal

    c. Otic

    d. Urethral

39. Which route of medication administration involves administering medication as a solution to the bladder?

    a. Ophthalmic

    b. Rectal

    c. Otic

    d. Bladder

40. Which route of medication administration involves administering medication as a solution into the spinal canal?

    a. Intrathecal

    b. Sublingual

    c. Intramuscular

    d. Topical

41. Which category of drugs relieves mild to severe pain?

    a.   Anesthetics

    b.   Antibiotics

    c.   Analgesics

    d.   Anticoagulants

42. Which category of drugs prevents sensation of pain?

    a.   Analgesics

    b.   Antibiotics

    c.   Anesthetics

    d.   Anticoagulants

43. Which category of drugs kills bacterial microorganisms?

    a.   Analgesics

    b.   Antibiotics

    c.   Anesthetics

    d.   Anticoagulants

44. Which category of drugs prevents blood from clotting?

    a.   Analgesics

    b.   Antibiotics

    c.   Anesthetics

    d.   Anticoagulants

45. Which category of drugs reduces blood pressure and increases urine output?

   a. Diuretics

   b. Vasoconstrictors

   c. Synergists

   d. Antagonists

46. Which category of drugs constricts blood vessels and increases blood pressure?

   a. Diuretics

   b. Vasoconstrictors

   c. Synergists

   d. Antagonists

47. Which term refers to two drugs working together?

   a. Synergist

   b. Antagonist

   c. Adverse reaction

   d. Volume

48. Which term refers to one drug decreasing the effect of another?

   a. Synergist

   b. Antagonist

   c. Adverse reaction

   d. Volume

49. Which term refers to undesirable effects of a particular drug?

    a. Synergist

    b. Antagonist

    c. Adverse reaction

    d. Volume

50. Which system of measurement is most commonly used in pharmacology and drug administration?

    a. Metric

    b. Apothecary

    c. Household

    d. Imperial

51. Which term refers to the amount of space a drug occupies?

    a. Weight

    b. Volume

    c. Liters

    d. Grams

52. Which unit of measurement is used to measure volumes in the metric system?

    a. Liters

    b. Grams

    c. Fluid ounces

    d. Fluid drams

53. Which unit of measurement is used to measure weight in the metric system?

    a. Liters

    b. Grams

    c. Fluid ounces

    d. Fluid drams

54. Which system of measurement uses fluid ounces and fluid drams?

    a. Metric

    b. Apothecary

    c. Household

    d. Imperial

55. Which term refers to heaviness?

    a. Weight

    b. Volume

    c. Liters

    d. Grams

56. Which category of drugs is used to treat high blood pressure?

    a. Analgesics

    b. Antibiotics

    c. Diuretics

    d. Anticoagulants

57. Which category of drugs is used to treat depression?

    a. Analgesics

    b. Antidepressants

    c. Anesthetics

    d. Anticoagulants

58. Which category of drugs is used to treat allergies?

    a. Analgesics

    b. Antibiotics

    c. Antihistamines

    d. Anticoagulants

59. Which term refers to the amount of drug given at one time?

    a. Dosage

    b. Frequency

    c. Route

    d. Duration

60. Which system of measurement uses teaspoons and tablespoons?

    a. Metric

    b. Apothecary

    c. Household

    d. Imperial

61. Which category of drugs is used to treat inflammation?

    a. Analgesics

    b. Antibiotics

    c. Antihistamines

    d. Anti-inflammatories

62. Which category of drugs is used to treat seizures?

    a. Analgesics

    b. Antibiotics

    c. Anticonvulsants

    d. Anticoagulants

63. Which term refers to the frequency of drug administration?

    a. Dosage

    b. Frequency

    c. Route

    d. Duration

64. Which system of measurement uses grains and scruples?

    a. Metric

    b. Apothecary

    c. Household

    d. Imperial

65. Which term refers to the method of drug administration?

    a.   Dosage

    b.   Frequency

    c.   Route

    d.   Duration

66. What is the Patient Care Partnership?

    a.   A guide for physicians only

    b.   A guide for patients only

    c.   A guide for both patients and physicians

    d.   A legal document for patients

67. What information should be provided to a patient before giving informed consent for a procedure or treatment?

    a.   Only the benefits of the procedure or treatment

    b.   Only the risks of the procedure or treatment

    c.   Both the risks and benefits of the procedure or treatment

    d.   No information is required for informed consent.

68. Can a patient refuse treatment, examination, or observation?

    a.   No, a patient cannot refuse any medical procedures.

    b.   Yes, but the patient will be charged a fee.

    c.   Yes, and the patient should be informed of the potential health effects.

    d.   No, a patient must comply with all medical procedures.

69. What is a patient's right regarding privacy and confidentiality?

    a. No privacy or confidentiality is guaranteed.

    b. Privacy is guaranteed, but confidentiality is not.

    c. Confidentiality is guaranteed, but privacy is not.

    d. Both privacy and confidentiality are guaranteed

70. Can a patient review their medical record without charge?

    a. No, a fee is always charged for reviewing medical records.

    b. Yes, but only if the patient is a family member.

    c. Yes, but only if the patient is retired.

    d. Yes, a patient can review their medical record without charge.

71. What is a patient's right regarding treatment without discrimination?

    a. Discrimination is allowed based on race, color, religion, gender, national origin, disability, or source of payment.

    b. Discrimination is allowed based on race, color, religion, or gender only.

    c. Discrimination is not allowed based on any of the listed factors.

    d. Discrimination is allowed based on source of payment only.

72. What is a patient's right regarding informed consent for an order not to resuscitate?

    a. No information is required for informed consent.

    b. Only the possible risks of the order not to resuscitate need to be provided.

    c. Only the possible benefits of the order not to resuscitate need to be provided.

    d. All the information needed to give informed consent, including the possible risks and benefits, needs to be provided.

73. Can a patient designate an individual to give informed consent for an order not to resuscitate?

    a. No, only the patient can give informed consent for an order not to resuscitate.

    b. Yes, but only if the patient is too ill to give informed consent.

    c. Yes, but only if the patient is not a family member.

    d. No, informed consent is not required for an order not to resuscitate.

74. What is a patient's right regarding obtaining a copy of their medical record?

    a. No patient has the right to obtain a copy of their medical record.

    b. A patient can obtain a copy of their medical record, but only if they pay a high fee.

    c. A patient can obtain a copy of their medical record, but only if they review it in the hospital.

    d. A patient can obtain a copy of their medical record for which the hospital can charge a reasonable fee.

75. What is a patient's right regarding being informed of the name and position of the doctor who will oversee their care in the hospital?

    a. No information is required to be provided about the overseeing doctor.

    b. Only the name of the overseeing doctor needs to be provided.

    c. Only the position of the overseeing doctor needs to be provided.

    d. Both the name and position of the overseeing doctor need to be provided

76. What is a patient's right regarding their participation in their own health care?

    a. Patients are not allowed to participate in their own health care.

    b. Patients are only allowed to participate in their own health care if they are a family member.

    c. Patients are actively encouraged to participate in their own health care.

    d. Patients are only allowed to participate in their own health care if they are not disabled.

77. What is a patient's right regarding being informed of the possible risks and benefits of a procedure or treatment?

    a. Patients do not have the right to be informed of the possible risks and benefits.

    b. Patients only have the right to be informed of the benefits.

    c. Patients only have the right to be informed of the risks.

    d. Patients have the right to be informed of both the possible risks and benefits.

78. What is a patient's right regarding their medical record?

    a. Patients do not have the right to review their medical record.

    b. Patients can review their medical record, but only if they pay a high fee.

    c. Patients can review their medical record without charge.

    d. Patients can only review their medical record if they are not a family member.

79. What is a patient's right regarding privacy while in the hospital?

    a. No privacy is guaranteed while in the hospital.

    b. Privacy is guaranteed, but only if the patient is not disabled.

    c. Privacy is guaranteed while in the hospital.

    d. Privacy is guaranteed, but only if the patient is not a family member.

80. What is a patient's right regarding confidentiality of their information and records?

    a. No confidentiality is guaranteed for a patient's information and records.

    b. Confidentiality is guaranteed, but only if the patient is not disabled.

    c. Confidentiality is guaranteed for all information and records regarding a patient's care.

    d. Confidentiality is guaranteed, but only if the patient is not a family member.

81. What is a patient's right regarding their pain management?

   a. Patients do not have the right to pain management.

   b. Patients have the right to pain management, but only if they are not disabled.

   c. Patients have the right to pain management.

   d. Patients have the right to pain management, but only if they are not a family member.

82. What is a patient's right regarding their right to refuse treatment?

   a. Patients do not have the right to refuse treatment.

   b. Patients have the right to refuse treatment, but only if they are not disabled.

   c. Patients have the right to refuse treatment.

   d. Patients have the right to refuse treatment, but only if they are not a family member.

83. What is a patient's right regarding their right to receive visitors?

   a. Patients do not have the right to receive visitors.

   b. Patients have the right to receive visitors, but only if they are not disabled.

   c. Patients have the right to receive visitors.

   d. Patients have the right to receive visitors, but only if they are not a family member.

84. What is a patient's right regarding their right to be involved in decisions about their care?

   a. Patients do not have the right to be involved in decisions about their care.

   b. Patients have the right to be involved in decisions about their care, but only if they are not disabled.

   c. Patients have the right to be involved in decisions about their care.

   d. Patients have the right to be involved in decisions about their care, but only if they are not a family member.

85. What is a patient's right regarding their right to receive information about their care?

   a. Patients do not have the right to receive information about their care.

   b. Patients have the right to receive information about their care, but only if they are not disabled.

   c. Patients have the right to receive information about their care.

   d. Patients have the right to receive information about their care, but only if they are not a family member.

86. What is a patient's right regarding their right to be treated with respect and dignity?

   a. Patients do not have the right to be treated with respect and dignity.

   b. Patients have the right to be treated with respect and dignity, but only if they are not disabled.

   c. Patients have the right to be treated with respect and dignity.

   d. Patients have the right to be treated with respect and dignity, but only if they are not a family member.

87. What is a patient's right regarding their right to have their cultural, psychosocial, and spiritual values respected?

   a. Patients do not have the right to have their cultural, psychosocial, and spiritual values respected.

   b. Patients have the right to have their cultural, psychosocial, and spiritual values respected, but only if they are not disabled.

   c. Patients have the right to have their cultural, psychosocial, and spiritual values respected.

   d. Patients have the right to have their cultural, psychosocial, and spiritual values respected, but only if they are not a family member.

88. What is a patient's right regarding their right to receive care in a safe environment?

    a. Patients do not have the right to receive care in a safe environment.

    b. Patients have the right to receive care in a safe environment, but only if they are not disabled.

    c. Patients have the right to receive care in a safe environment.

    d. Patients have the right to receive care in a safe environment, but only if they are not a family member.

89. What is a patient's right regarding their right to have their pain assessed and managed?

    a. Patients do not have the right to have their pain assessed and managed.

    b. Patients have the right to have their pain assessed and managed, but only if they are not disabled.

    c. Patients have the right to have their pain assessed and managed.

    d. Patients have the right to have their pain assessed and managed, but only if they are not a family member.

90. What is a patient's right regarding their right to receive care without discrimination?

    a. Patients do not have the right to receive care without discrimination.

    b. Patients have the right to receive care without discrimination, but only if they are not disabled.

    c. Patients have the right to receive care without discrimination.

    d. Patients have the right to receive care without discrimination, but only if they are not a family member.

91. What is a patient's right regarding their right to privacy and confidentiality?

    a. Patients do not have the right to privacy and confidentiality.

    b. Patients have the right to privacy and confidentiality, but only if they are not disabled.

    c. Patients have the right to privacy and confidentiality.

    d. Patients have the right to privacy and confidentiality, but only if they are not a family member.

92. What is a patient's right regarding their right to access their medical records?

    a. Patients do not have the right to access their medical records.

    b. Patients have the right to access their medical records, but only if they are not disabled.

    c. Patients have the right to access their medical records.

    d. Patients have the right to access their medical records, but only if they are not a family member.

93. What is a patient's right regarding their right to receive information about their diagnosis, treatment, and prognosis?

    a. Patients do not have the right to receive information about their diagnosis, treatment, and prognosis.

    b. Patients have the right to receive information about their diagnosis, treatment, and prognosis, but only if they are not disabled.

    c. Patients have the right to receive information about their diagnosis, treatment, and prognosis.

    d. Patients have the right to receive information about their diagnosis, treatment, and prognosis, but only if they are not a family member.

94. What is a patient's right regarding their right to participate in research studies?

   a. Patients do not have the right to participate in research studies.

   b. Patients have the right to participate in research studies, but only if they are not disabled.

   c. Patients have the right to participate in research studies.

   d. Patients have the right to participate in research studies, but only if they are not a family member.

95. What is a patient's right regarding their right to receive care that is free from restraints or seclusion?

   a. Patients do not have the right to receive care that is free from restraints or seclusion.

   b. Patients have the right to receive care that is free from restraints or seclusion, but only if they are not disabled.

   c. Patients have the right to receive care that is free from restraints or seclusion.

   d. Patients have the right to receive care that is free from restraints or seclusion, but only if they are not a family member.

96. What is a patient's right regarding their right to make decisions about their care?

   a. Patients do not have the right to make decisions about their care.

   b. Patients have the right to make decisions about their care, but only if they are not disabled.

   c. Patients have the right to make decisions about their care.

   d. Patients have the right to make decisions about their care, but only if they are not a family member.

97. What is a patient's right regarding their right to receive information about their treatment options?

   a. Patients do not have the right to receive information about their treatment options.

   b. Patients have the right to receive information about their treatment options, but only if they are not disabled.

   c. Patients have the right to receive information about their treatment options.

   d. Patients have the right to receive information about their treatment options, but only if they are not a family member.

98. What is a patient's right regarding their right to refuse treatment?

   a. Patients do not have the right to refuse treatment.

   b. Patients have the right to refuse treatment, but only if they are not disabled.

   c. Patients have the right to refuse treatment.

   d. Patients have the right to refuse treatment, but only if they are not a family member.

99. What is a patient's right regarding their right to have a family member or representative involved in their care?

   a. Patients do not have the right to have a family member or representative involved in their care.

   b. Patients have the right to have a family member or representative involved in their care, but only if they are not disabled.

   c. Patients have the right to have a family member or representative involved in their care.

   d. Patients have the right to have a family member or representative involved in their care, but only if they are not a family member.

100. What is a patient's right regarding their right to receive information about hospital charges and payment methods?

   a. Patients do not have the right to receive information about hospital charges and payment methods.

   b. Patients have the right to receive information about hospital charges and payment methods, but only if they are not disabled.

   c. Patients have the right to receive information about hospital charges and payment methods.

   d. Patients have the right to receive information about hospital charges and payment methods, but only if they are not a family member.

PART-FIVE

ANSWER TO MEDICAL ASSISTANT QUESTIONS

1. **Answer C**

   12-20 per minute

2. **Answer A**

   By counting the number of respirations per minute

3. **Answer C**

   A temporary complete absence of breathing

4. **Answer B**

   A respiration rate of greater than 40/min

5. **Answer A**

   A decrease in number of respirations

6. **Answer A**

   The measurement of the amount of force exerted by the blood on the peripheral arterial.

7. **Answer A.**

   Systole and diastole

8. **Answer A**

   120/80 mmHg

9. **Answer A**

   Signs of abnormality in beats

10. **Answer A**

    An indication of valvular heart disease

11. **Answer C**

Count the number of respirations for 30 seconds and multiply by two.

12. **Answer A**

A reduction in the stimuli to the respiratory centers of the brain

13. **Answer A**

Hysteria

14. **Answer A**

Decrease in number of respirations during sleep.

15. **Answer A**

Millimeters of mercury (mmHg)

16. **Answer C**

To measure the amount of force exerted by the blood on the peripheral arterial walls.

17. **Answer A**

Systolic is the highest amount of pressure exerted during the cardiac cycle, while diastolic is the lowest amount of pressure.

18. **Answer C**

30-35 per minute

19. **Answer C**

Respiratory disease

20. **Answer A**

A reduction in the stimuli to the respiratory centers of the brain

21. **Answer B**

Sublingual: Medication is placed under the tongue until it dissolves.

22. Answer C

Intramuscular: Medication is injected into the muscle.

23. Answer C

Topical: Drug is rubbed into, patted on, sprayed on, or swabbed on.

24. Answer A

Ophthalmic: Instillation of medications into the eyes.

25. Answer B

Rectal: Suppository is inserted into the rectum, or a solution is administered as an enema.

26. Answer D

Vaginal: A solution is administered as a douche.

27. Answer B

Subcutaneous: Medication is injected into the subcutaneous layer of the skin at a 45-degree angle.

28. Answer A

Inhalation: Drug is inhaled to achieve local effects within the respiratory tract.

29. Answer A

Intradermal: Medication is injected between the upper layers of the skin at a 15-degree angle.

30. Answer C

Otic: Instillations of medications (usually drops) into the ear.

31. Answer C

Transdermal: Route is typically in the patch form, provides continuous absorption and effects that last over many hours.

32. Answer C

Intramuscular: Medication is injected into the muscle at a 90-degree angle and aspirated.

33. Answer B

Rectal: Administering medication as a solution into the rectum.

34. Answer B

Sublingual: Asking the patient to place medication between their cheek and gum until it dissolves.

35. Answer D

Vaginal: Administering medication as a solution to the vagina.

36. Answer D

Rectal: Administering medication as an enema.

37. Answer A

Inhalation: Administering medication as a spray or mist into the nose.

38. Answer D

Urethral: Administering medication as a solution into the urethra.

39. Answer D

Bladder: Administering medication as a solution to the bladder.

40. Answer A

Intrathecal: Administering medication as a solution into the spinal canal.

41. Answer: C

Analgesics

42. Answer: C

Anesthetics

43. Answer: B

Antibiotics

44. Answer: D

Anticoagulants

45. Answer: A

Diuretics

46. Answer: B

Vasoconstrictors

47. Answer: A

Synergist

48. Answer: B

Antagonist

49. Answer: C

Adverse reaction

50. Answer: A

Metric

51. Answer: B

Volume

52. Answer: A

Liters

53. Answer: B

Grams

54. Answer: A

Weight

55. Answer: B

Apothecary

56. Answer C

Diuretics: Medications that are used to treat high blood pressure by increasing urine output and reducing fluid buildup.

57. Answer B

Antidepressants: Medications that are used to treat depression by altering brain chemistry.

58. Answer C

Antihistamines: Medications that are used to treat allergies by blocking the effects of histamine.

59. Answer A

Dosage: The amount of a drug that is given at one time.

60. Answer C

Household: A system of measurement that is used for common household items, such as teaspoons and tablespoons.

61. Answer D

Anti-inflammatories: Medications that are used to treat inflammation by reducing swelling and pain.

62. Answer C

Anticonvulsants: Medications that are used to treat seizures by stabilizing brain activity.

63. Answer B

Frequency: The number of times a drug is given in a certain period of time.

64. Answer B

Apothecary: A system of measurement that is used for medications and is based on grains and scruples.

65. Answer C

Route: The method of drug administration, such as oral, intravenous, or topical.

66. Answer: C

A guide for both patients and physicians

67. Answer: C

Both the risks and benefits of the procedure or treatment

68. Answer: C

Yes, and the patient should be informed of the potential health effects.

69. Answer: D

Both privacy and confidentiality are guaranteed

70. Answer: D

Yes, a patient can review their medical record without charge.

71. Answer: C

Discrimination is not allowed based on any of the listed factors.

72. Answer: D

All the information needed to give informed consent, including the possible risks and benefits, needs to be provided.

73. Answer: B

Yes, but only if the patient is too ill to give informed consent.

74. Answer: D

A patient can obtain a copy of their medical record for which the hospital can charge a reasonable fee

75. Answer: D

Both the name and position of the overseeing doctor need to be provided

76. Answer: C

Patients are actively encouraged to participate in their own health care.

77. Answer: D

Patients have the right to be informed of both the possible risks and benefits.

78. Answer: C

Patients can review their medical record without charge.

79. Answer: C

Privacy is guaranteed while in the hospital.

80. Answer: C

Confidentiality is guaranteed for all information and records regarding a patient's care.

81. Answer: C

Patients have the right to pain management.

82. Answer: C

Patients have the right to refuse treatment.

83. Answer: C

Patients have the right to receive visitors.

84. Answer: C

Patients have the right to be involved in decisions about their care.

85. Answer: C

Patients have the right to receive information about their care.

86. Answer: C

Patients have the right to be treated with respect and dignity.

87. Answer: C

Patients have the right to have their cultural, psychosocial, and spiritual values respected.

88. Answer: C

Patients have the right to receive care in a safe environment.

89. Answer: C

Patients have the right to have their pain assessed and managed.

90. Answer: C

Patients have the right to receive care without discrimination.

91. Answer: C

Patients have the right to privacy and confidentiality.

92. Answer: C

Patients have the right to access their medical records.

93. Answer: C

Patients have the right to receive information about their diagnosis, treatment, and prognosis.

94. Answer: C

Patients have the right to participate in research studies.

95. Answer: C

Patients have the right to receive care that is free from restraints or seclusion.

96. Answer: C

Patients have the right to make decisions about their care.

97. Answer: C

Patients have the right to receive information about their treatment options.

98. Answer: C

Patients have the right to refuse treatment.

99. Answer: C

Patients have the right to receive information about hospital charges and payment methods.

100. Answer: C

Patients have the right to have a family member or representative involved in their care.

MEDICAL ASSISTANT CERTIFICATION
EXAMINATION STUDY GUIDE
PART-SIX

1. What is the purpose of combining vowels in a medical term?

    a. To make the word easier to say

    b. To change the meaning of the word

    c. To indicate the location of the body part

    d. To indicate the type of medical procedure

2. Which term refers to the front part of the body?

    a. Ventral

    b. Dorsal

    c. Anterior

    d. Posterior

3. What is the purpose of a prefix in a medical term?

    a. To indicate the location of the body part

    b. To make the word easier to say

    c. To change the meaning of the word

    d. To indicate the type of medical procedure

4. Which term refers to the back part of the body?

    a. Ventral

    b. Dorsal

    c. Anterior

    d. Posterior

5. What is the purpose of a suffix in a medical term?

    a. To indicate the location of the body part

    b. To make the word easier to say

    c. To change the meaning of the word

    d. To indicate the type of medical procedure

6. Which term refers to the side of the body?

    a. Medial

    b. Lateral

    c. Proximal

    d. Distal

7. Which plane divides the body into front and back portions?

    a. Ventral plane

    b. Dorsal plane

    c. Anterior plane

    d. Frontal plane

8. . Which term refers to the upper portion of the body?

    a. Ventral

    b. Dorsal

    c. Anterior

    d. Superior

9. Which term refers to the lower portion of the body?

    a. Ventral

    b. Dorsal

    c. Anterior

    d. Inferior

10. Which term refers to a structure that is closest to the point of origin?

    a. Proximal

    b. Distal

    c. Medial

    d. Lateral

11. Which term refers to a structure that is far from the point of origin?

    a. Proximal

    b. Distal

    c. Medial

    d. Lateral

12. Which term refers to a structure that is towards the midline of the body?

    a. Medial

    b. Lateral

    c. Proximal

    d. Distal

13. Which plane divides the body into upper and lower portions?

    a. Ventral plane

    b. Dorsal plane

    c. Anterior plane

    d. Transverse plane

14. Which term refers to a structure that is below another structure?

    a. Superior

    b. Inferior

    c. Medial

    d. Lateral

15. Which term refers to a structure that is towards the back part of the body?

    a. Ventral

    b. Dorsal

    c. Anterior

    d. Posterior

16. Which term refers to a structure that is away from the surface?

    a. Anterior

    b. Posterior

    c. Deep

    d. Proximal

17. Which term refers to the near the point of attachment to the trunk or near the beginning of a structure?

    a. Proximal

    b. Distal

    c. Medial

    d. Lateral

18. . Which term refers to the far from the point of attachment to the trunk or far from the beginning of a structure?

    a. Proximal

    b. Distal

    c. Medial

    d. Lateral

19. Which term refers to the front surface of the body?

    a. Ventral

    b. Dorsal

    c. Anterior

    d. Posterior

20. Which term refers to the back side of the body?

    a. Ventral

    b. Dorsal

    c. Anterior

    d. Posterior

21. . Which term refers to the division of a medical term that comes before the root word?

    a.   Suffix

    b.   Combining vowel

    c.   Prefix

    d.   Body direction term

22. Which term refers to the division of a medical term that comes after the root word?

    a.   Suffix

    b.   Combining vowel

    c.   Prefix

    d.   Body direction term

23. Which term refers to the division of a medical term that makes the word easier to say?

    a.   Suffix

    b.   Combining vowel

    c.   Prefix

    d.   Body direction term

24. Which term refers to the division of a medical term that indicates the location of the body part?

    a.   Suffix

    b.   Combining vowel

    c.   Prefix

    d.   Body direction term

25. Which term refers to the front part of the body?

    a.   Ventral

    b.   Dorsal

    c.   Anterior

    d.   Posterior

26. Which term refers to the back part of the body?

    a.   Ventral

    b.   Dorsal

    c.   Anterior

    d.   Posterior

27. . Which term refers to a structure that is towards the midline of the body?

    a.   Medial

    b.   Lateral

    c.   Proximal

    d.   Distal

28. Which term refers to a structure that is away from the midline of the body?

    a.   Medial

    b.   Lateral

    c.   Proximal

    d.   Distal

29. . Which term refers to a structure that is closest to the point of origin?

    a. Proximal

    b. Distal

    c. Medial

    d. Lateral

30. Which term refers to a structure that is far from the point of origin?

    a. Proximal

    b. Distal

    c. Medial

    d. Lateral

31. . Which term refers to a structure that is below another structure?

    a. Superior

    b. Inferior

    c. Medial

    d. Lateral

32. Which term refers to a structure that is above another structure?

    a. Superior

    b. Inferior

    c. Medial

    d. Lateral

33. Which plane divides the body into front and back portions?

    a. Ventral plane

    b. Dorsal plane

    c. Anterior plane

    d. Frontal plane

34. Which plane divides the body into upper and lower portions?

    a. Ventral plane

    b. Dorsal plane

    c. Anterior plane

    d. Transverse plane

35. Which term refers to a structure that is towards the front part of the body?

    a. Ventral

    b. Dorsal

    c. Anterior

    d. Posterior

36. Which term refers to a structure that is towards the back part of the body?

    a. Ventral

    b. Dorsal

    c. Anterior

    d. Posterior

37. Which term refers to a structure that is towards the surface of the body?

   a. Anterior

   b. Posterior

   c. Superficial

   d. Deep

38. Which term refers to a structure that is away from the surface of the body?

   a. Anterior

   b. Posterior

   c. Superficial

   d. Deep

39. Which term refers to the division of a medical term that connects the root word to the suffix?

   a. Suffix

   b. Combining vowel

   c. Prefix

   d. Body direction term

40. Which term refers to the division of a medical term that indicates a condition or disease?

   a. Suffix

   b. Combining vowel

   c. Prefix

   d. Body direction term

41. . Which term refers to the division of a medical term that indicates a procedure or action?

    a. Suffix

    b. Combining vowel

    c. Prefix

    d. Body direction term

42. Which term refers to the division of a medical term that indicates a location or direction?

    a. Suffix

    b. Combining vowel

    c. Prefix

    d. Body direction term

43. Which term refers to the division of a medical term that indicates a number or measurement?

    a. Suffix

    b. Combining vowel

    c. Prefix

    d. Body direction term

44. Which term refers to the division of a medical term that indicates a time or frequency?

    a. Suffix

    b. Combining vowel

    c. Prefix

    d. Body direction term

45. Which term refers to the division of a medical term that indicates a quality or state?

    a. Suffix

    b. Combining vowel

    c. Prefix

    d. Body direction term

46. Which term refers to the division of a medical term that indicates a body system or part?

    a. Suffix

    b. Combining vowel

    c. Prefix

    d. Body direction term

47. Which term refers to the division of a medical term that indicates a drug or medication?

    a. Suffix

    b. Combining vowel

    c. Prefix

    d. Body direction term

48. . Which term refers to the division of a medical term that indicates a symptom or sign?

    a. Suffix

    b. Combining vowel

    c. Prefix

    d. Body direction term

49. Which term refers to the division of a medical term that indicates a surgical instrument?

   a. Suffix

   b. Combining vowel

   c. Prefix

   d. Body direction term

50. Which term refers to the division of a medical term that indicates a body cavity or space?

   a. Suffix

   b. Combining vowel

   c. Prefix

   d. Body direction term

51. What is the term used for lying on the side?

   a. Supine position

   b. Prone position

   c. Lateral recumbent position

   d. Normal anatomic position

52. Which type of joint is slightly moveable and joined together by cartilage?

   a. Synovial joint

   b. Diarthrosis joint

   c. Amphiarthrosis joint

   d. Synarthrosis joint

53. What is the term used for decreasing the angle of a joint?

    a.   Extension

    b.   Flexion

    c.   Abduction

    d.   Adduction

54. Which body position involves standing with arms lank and palms forward?

    a.   Supine position

    b.   Prone position

    c.   Lateral recumbent position

    d.   Normal anatomic position

55. Which type of joint is surrounded by joint capsules and has sacs of fluid called bursae?

    a.   Synovial joint

    b.   Diarthrosis joint

    c.   Amphiarthrosis joint

    d.   Synarthrosis joint

56. . What is the term used for movement towards the midline of the body?

    a.   Extension

    b.   Flexion

    c.   Abduction

    d.   Adduction

57. Which body position involves lying on the back?

    a. Supine position

    b. Prone position

    c. Lateral recumbent position

    d. Normal anatomic position

58. Which type of joint is found in the skull and allows for very little movement?

    a. Synovial joint

    b. Diarthrosis joint

    c. Amphiarthrosis joint

    d. Synarthrosis joint

59. What is the term used for increasing the angle of a joint?

    a. Extension

    b. Flexion

    c. Abduction

    d. Adduction

60. Which type of joint is found in the spine and allows for limited movement?

    a. Synovial joint

    b. Diarthrosis joint

    c. Amphiarthrosis joint

    d. Synarthrosis joint

61. What is the term used for movement away from the midline of the body?

    a. Extension

    b. Flexion

    c. Abduction

    d. Adduction

62. Which body position involves lying face down?

    a. Supine position

    b. Prone position

    c. Lateral recumbent position

    d. Normal anatomic position

63. Which type of joint is found in the shoulder and hip and allows for a wide range of movement?

    a. Synovial joint

    b. Diarthrosis joint

    c. Amphiarthrosis joint

    d. Synarthrosis joint

64. What is the term used for rotating a joint towards the midline of the body?

    a. Internal rotation

    b. External rotation

    c. Abduction

    d. Adduction

65. Which type of joint is found in the elbow and knee and allows for movement in one plane?

    a.   Synovial joint

    b.   Diarthrosis joint

    c.   Amphiarthrosis joint

    d.   Synarthrosis joint

66. What is the term used for rotating a joint away from the midline of the body?

    a.   Internal rotation

    b.   External rotation

    c.   Abduction

    d.   Adduction

67. Which body position involves lying on the side?

    a.   Supine position

    b.   Prone position

    c.   Lateral recumbent position

    d.   Normal anatomic position

68. Which type of joint is found in the wrist and ankle and allows for movement in multiple planes?

    a.   Synovial joint

    b.   Diarthrosis joint

    c.   Amphiarthrosis joint

    d.   Synarthrosis joint

69. What is the term used for bending a joint?

    a. Extension

    b. Flexion

    c. Abduction

    d. Adduction

70. Which type of joint is found in the skull and allows for some movement?

    a. Synovial joint

    b. Diarthrosis joint

    c. Amphiarthrosis joint

    d. Synarthrosis joint

71. What is the difference between criminal and civil laws?

    a. Criminal laws are concerned with relationships between people, while civil laws are concerned with offenses against the public.

    b. Criminal laws are concerned with offenses against the public, while civil laws are concerned with relationships between people.

    c. Criminal laws are concerned with intentional wrongs, while civil laws are concerned with unintentional wrongs.

    d. Criminal laws are concerned with unintentional wrongs, while civil laws are concerned with intentional wrongs.

72. What is a tort?

    a. A criminal offense

    b. A civil offense

    c. A breach of confidentiality

    d. A subpoena

73. What does it mean to be liable?

   a. To be held accountable under law

   b. To commit an intentional tort

   c. To breach confidentiality

   d. To commit malpractice

74. What is breach of confidentiality?

   a. Making false statements to a third person

   b. Injuring a person's name and reputation

   c. Violating a person's right to privacy

   d. Revealing information about a patient without consent

75. What is negligence?

   a. An intentional wrong

   b. A breach of confidentiality

   c. A civil offense

   d. An unintentional wrong

76. What is malpractice?

   a. An intentional wrong

   b. A breach of confidentiality

   c. A civil offense

   d. Negligence by a professional person

77. . What is malfeasance?

    a. An intentional wrong

    b. A breach of confidentiality

    c. A civil offense

    d. An unintentional wrong

78. What is defamation?

    a. Revealing information about a patient without consent

    b. Injuring a person's name and reputation by making false statements to a third person

    c. Violating a person's right to privacy

    d. Saying or doing something to trick, fool or deceive a person.

79. What is the difference between libel and slander?

    a. Libel is making false statements orally, while slander is making false statements in print, writing or through pictures.

    b. Libel is a civil offense, while slander is a criminal offense.

    c. Libel is an intentional wrong, while slander is an unintentional wrong.

    d. Libel is making false statements in print, writing or through pictures, while slander is making false statements orally.

80. What is fraud?

    a. Revealing information about a patient without consent

    b. Injuring a person's name and reputation by making false statements to a third person

    c. Saying or doing something to trick, fool or deceive a person.

    d. Violating a person's right to privacy

81. What is assault?

    a. Touching a person's body without their consent

    b. Intentionally attempting to touch or threaten a person's body without their consent.

    c. Revealing information about a patient without consent

    d. Injuring a person's name and reputation by making false statements to a third person

82. What is a battery?

    a. Touching a person's body without their consent

    b. Intentionally attempting to touch or threaten a person's body without their consent.

    c. Revealing information about a patient without consent

    d. Injuring a person's name and reputation by making false statements to a third person

83. What is a misdemeanor?

    a. A crime punishable by more than one year

    b. A civil offense

    c. A crime punishable by one year or less

    d. An intentional wrong

84. . What is a felony?

    a. A crime punishable by one year or less

    b. A civil offense

    c. An unintentional wrong

    d. A crime punishable by more than one year

85. What is a subpoena?

   a. An order issued by the court to obtain evidence.

   b. A civil offense

   c. An intentional wrong

   d. A breach of confidentiality

86. . What is invasion of privacy?

   a. Revealing information about a patient without consent

   b. Injuring a person's name and reputation by making false statements to a third person

   c. Violating a person's right not to have their private affairs exposed.

   d. Saying or doing something to trick, fool or deceive a person.

87. What is the difference between intentional and unintentional torts?

   a. Intentional torts are acts that are meant to be harmful, while unintentional torts are acts that are not meant to be harmful.

   b. Intentional torts are civil offenses, while unintentional torts are criminal offenses.

   c. Intentional torts are acts that are not meant to be harmful, while unintentional torts are acts that are meant to be harmful.

   d. Intentional torts are criminal offenses, while unintentional torts are civil offenses.

88. What is the difference between libel and slander?

   a. Libel is an unintentional wrong, while slander is an intentional wrong.

   b. Libel is making false statements in print, writing or through pictures, while slander is making false statements orally.

   c. Libel is a criminal offense, while slander is a civil offense.

   d. Libel is making false statements orally, while slander is making false statements in print, writing or through pictures.

89. What is the difference between malpractice and malfeasance?

    a. Malpractice is an intentional wrong, while malfeasance is an unintentional wrong.

    b. Malpractice is negligence by a professional person, while malfeasance is an affirmative act that is illegal or wrongful.

    c. Malpractice is a civil offense, while malfeasance is a criminal offense.

    d. Malpractice is a breach of confidentiality, while malfeasance is an invasion of privacy.

90. What is the difference between assault and battery?

    a. Assault is touching a person's body without their consent, while battery is intentionally attempting to touch or threaten a person's body without their consent.

    b. Assault is an unintentional wrong, while battery is an intentional wrong.

    c. Assault is intentionally attempting to touch or threaten a person's body without their consent, while battery is touching a person's body without their consent.

    d. Assault is a civil offense, while battery is a criminal offense.

91. What is a medical record?

    a. A written account of a person's condition and response to treatment and care

    b. A list of medications prescribed to a patient.

    c. A summary of a patient's medical history

    d. A report of a patient's vital signs

92. What are the parts of a medical record?

    a. Admission sheet, nursing history, graphic sheet, progress notes, flow sheets

    b. Prescription list, lab results, imaging reports, discharge summary

    c. Patient demographics, insurance information, billing records

    d. Physician notes, consultation reports, surgical reports

93. What is the difference between reporting and recording in patient care?

    a.   Reporting is the written account of care and observations, while recording is the oral account of care.

    b.   Reporting is the oral account of care and observations, while recording is the written account of care.

    c.   Reporting and recording are the same thing.

    d.   Reporting and recording are not necessarily in-patient care.

94. What is the difference between objective and subjective data in patient assessment?

    a.   Objective data is information that is heard, felt, or smelled, while subjective data are things a person tells you about that you cannot observe through your senses.

    b.   Objective data is things a person tells you about that you cannot observe through your senses, while subjective data is information that is heard, felt, or smelled.

    c.   Objective and subjective data are the same thing.

    d.   Objective and subjective data are not necessarily in-patient assessment.

95. What is acute pain?

    a.   Pain that lasts longer possible for a lifetime

    b.   Pain that occurs after an amputation

    c.   Pain that lessens with treatment

    d.   Pain that is psychological in nature

96. What is chronic pain?

    a.   Pain that lasts longer possible for a lifetime

    b.   Pain that occurs after an amputation

    c.   Pain that lessens with treatment

    d.   Pain that is psychological in nature

97. What is physical pain?

    a. Pain that lasts longer possible for a lifetime

    b. Pain that occurs after an amputation

    c. Pain that lessens with treatment

    d. Pain is a sign that something is wrong.

98. What is psychological pain?

    a. Pain that lasts longer possible for a lifetime

    b. Pain that occurs after an amputation

    c. Pain that lessens with treatment

    d. Pain that could lead to disorders such as depression, PTSD, or an anxiety disorder.

99. What is phantom pain?

    a. Pain that lasts longer possible for a lifetime

    b. Pain that occurs after an amputation

    c. Pain that lessens with treatment

    d. Pain that is psychological in nature

100. What is nursing history in a medical record?

    a. A written account of a person's condition and response to treatment and care

    b. A summary of a patient's medical history

    c. A report of a patient's vital signs

    d. A record of a patient's nursing care plan

PART-SIX
ANSWER TO MEDICAL ASSISTANT QUESTIONS

1. Answer A

   To make the word easier to say

2. Answer A

   Ventral

3. Answer B

   To make the word easier to say

4. Answer B

   Dorsal

5. Answer C

   To change the meaning of the word

6. Answer B

   Lateral

7. Answer D

   Frontal plane

8. Answer D

   Superior

9. Answer D

   Inferior

10. Answer A

    Proximal

11. Answer B

    Distal

12. Answer A

    Medial

13. Answer D

    Transverse plane

14. Answer B

    Inferior

15. Answer D

    Posterior

16. Answer C

    Deep

17. Answer A

    Proximal

18. Answer B

    Distal

19. Answer C

    Anterior

20. Answer B

    Dorsal

21. Answer C

    Prefix

22. Answer A

    Suffix

23. Answer B

    Combining vowel

24. Answer D

    Body direction term

25. Answer A

    Ventral

26. Answer B

    Dorsal

27. Answer A

    Medial

28. Answer B

    Lateral

29. Answer A

    Proximal

30. Answer B

    Distal

31. Answer B

    Inferior

32. Answer A

    Superior

33. Answer D

    Frontal plane

34. Answer D

    Transverse plane

35. Answer C

    Anterior

36. Answer B

   Dorsal

37. Answer C

   Superficial

38. Answer D

   Deep

39. Answer B

   Combining vowel

40. Answer A

   Suffix

41. Answer A

   Suffix

42. Answer A

   Suffix

43. Answer A

   Suffix

44. Answer A

   Suffix

45. Answer A

   Suffix

46. Answer A

   Suffix

47. Answer A

   Suffix

48. Answer A

   Suffix

49. Answer A

   Suffix

50. Answer A

   Suffix

51. Answer: C

   Lateral recumbent position

52. Answer: C

   Amphiarthrosis join

53. Answer: B

   Flexion

54. Answer: D

Normal anatomic position

55. Answer: A

Synovial joint

56. Answer: D

Adduction

57. Answer: A

Supine position

58. Answer: D

Synarthrosis joint

59. Answer: A

Extension

60. Answer: C

Amphiarthrosis joint

61. Answer: C

Abduction

62. Answer: B

Prone position

63. Answer: A

Synovial joint

64. Answer: A

Internal rotation

65. Answer: B

Diarthrosis joint

66. Answer: B

External rotation

67. Answer: C

Lateral recumbent position

68. Answer: A

Synovial joint

69. Answer: B

Flexion

70. Answer: C

Amphiarthrosis joint

71. Answer: B

Criminal laws are concerned with offenses against the public, while civil laws are

concerned with relationships between people.

72. Answer: B

A civil offense

73. Answer: A

To be held accountable under law

74. Answer: D

Revealing information about a patient without consent

75. Answer: D

An unintentional wrong

76. Answer: D

Negligence by a professional person

77. Answer: A

intentional wrong

78. Answer: B

Injuring a person's name and reputation by making false statements to a third person

79. Answer: D

Libel is making false statements in print, writing or through pictures, while slander is making false

statements orally.

80. Answer: C

Saying or doing something to trick, fool or deceive a person.

81. Answer: B

Intentionally attempting to touch or threaten a person's body without their consent.

82. Answer: A

Touching a person's body without their consent

83. Answer: C

A crime punishable by one year or less

84. Answer: D

A crime punishable by more than one year

85. Answer: A

An order issued by the court to obtain evidence.

86. Answer: C

Violating a person's right not to have their private affairs exposed.

87. Answer: A

Intentional torts are acts that are meant to be harmful, while unintentional torts are acts that are

not meant to be harmful.

88. Answer: B

Libel is making false statements in print, writing or through pictures, while slander is making false

statements orally.

89. Answer: B

Malpractice is negligence by a professional person, while malfeasance is an

affirmative act that is illegal or wrongful.

90. Answer: C

Assault is intentionally attempting to touch or threaten a person's body without

their consent, while the battery is touching a person's body without their consent.

91. Answer: A

A written account of a person's condition and response to treatment and care

92. Answer: A

Admission sheet, nursing history, graphic sheet, progress notes, flow sheets

93. Answer: B

Reporting is the oral account of care and observations, while recording is the written account of

care

94. Answer: A

Objective data is information that is heard, felt, or smelled, while subjective data are things a person.

tells you about that you cannot observe through your senses

95. Answer: C

Pain that lessens with treatment

96. Answer: A

   Pain that lasts longer possible for a lifetime

97. Answer: D

   Pain is a sign that something is wrong.

98. Answer: D

   Pain that could lead to disorders such as depression, PTSD, or an anxiety disorder.

99. Answer: B

   Pain that occurs after an amputation

100. Answer: D

   A record of a patient's nursing care plan

MEDICAL ASSISTANT CERTIFICATION
EXAMINATION STUDY GUIDE
PART-SEVEN

1. What effect does calorie-rich food or drinks have on body temperature?

    a. Decrease

    b. Increase

    c. No effect

    d. Cannot be determined.

2. What effect do calorie-restricted diets have on body temperature?

    a. Decrease

    b. Increase

    c. No effect

    d. Cannot be determined.

3. What effect does alcohol consumption have on body temperature?

    a. Increase during the day and night.

    b. Decrease during the day and night.

    c. Increase during the night and decrease during the day.

    d. Decrease during the night and increase during the day.

4. What effect does physical activity have on body temperature?

    a. Decrease

    b. Increase

    c. No effect

    d. Cannot be determined.

5. Who can reach higher temperatures with minimum physical activity?

    a. Adults

    b. Children

    c. Both adults and children

    d. Cannot be determined.

6. What effect does a higher level of excitement have on body temperature?

    a. Decrease

    b. Increase

    c. No effect

    d. Cannot be determined.

7. What effect does sleep have on body temperature?

    a. Increase throughout the night.

    b. Decrease throughout the night.

    c. No effect

    d. Cannot be determined.

8. What effect does short-term sleep deprivation have on body temperature?

    a. Increase at night.

    b. Decrease at night.

    c. No effect

    d. Cannot be determined.

9. What effect does long-term sleep deprivation have on body temperature?

    a. Increase at night.

    b. Decrease at night.

    c. No effect

    d. Cannot be determined.

10. What factors can affect body temperature besides sleep patterns?

    a. Shift work, waking up at unusual times, and jet lag.

    b. Diet and exercise

    c. Emotional or mental state of mind

    d. All of the above

11. What effect does poor sleep quality or insomnia have on body temperature?

    a. Increase

    b. Decrease

    c. No effect

    d. Cannot be determined.

12. What effect do changes to shift work have on body temperature?

    a. Increase

    b. Decrease

    c. No effect

    d. Cannot be determined.

13. What effect does wake up at unusual times have on body temperature?

    a.   Increase

    b.   Decrease

    c.   No effect

    d.   Cannot be determined.

14. What effect does jet lag have on body temperature?

    a.   Increase

    b.   Decrease

    c.   No effect

    d.   Cannot be determined.

15. What is the general trend of body temperature at night?

    a.   Increase

    b.   Decrease

    c.   No effect

    d.   Cannot be determined.

16. What effect does sustaining physical activity have on body temperature in adults?

    a. Decrease

    b. Increase

    c. No effect

    d. Cannot be determined.

17. What effect does sustaining physical activity have on body temperature in children?

    a. Decrease

    b. Increase

    c. No effect

    d. Cannot be determined.

18. What effect does emotional or mental stress have on body temperature?

    a. Decrease

    b. Increase

    c. No effect

    d. Cannot be determined.

19. What effect does short-term sleep deprivation have on body temperature?

    a. Increase at night.

    b. Decrease at night.

    c. Increase during the day.

    d. Decrease during the day.

20. What effect does long-term sleep deprivation have on body temperature?

    a. Increase at night.

    b. Decrease at night.

    c. Increase during the day.

    d. Decrease during the day.

21. Which body part is typically used for oral temperature measurement?

    a. Anus

    b. Ear

    c. Mouth

    d. Vagina

22. Which body part is typically used for rectal temperature measurement?

   a. Anus

   b. Ear

   c. Mouth

   d. Vagina

23. Which body part is typically used for tympanic temperature measurement?

   a. Anus

   b. Ear

   c. Mouth

   d. Vagina

24. Which body part is typically used for axillary temperature measurement?

   a. Anus

   b. Ear

   c. Mouth

   d. Under the arm

25. Which body part is typically used for vaginal temperature measurement?

    a.   Anus

    b.   Ear

    c.   Mouth

    d.   Vagina

26. What is the typical daytime temperature reading for rectal, vaginal, and tympanic

measurements in healthy adults?

    a.   97.6°F

    b.   98.2°F

    c.   99.7°F

    d.   Cannot be determined.

27. What is the typical daytime temperature reading for oral measurements in healthy adults?

    a.   97.6°F

    b.   98.2°F

    c.   99.7°F

    d.   Cannot be determined.

28. What is the typical daytime temperature reading for axillary measurements in healthy adults?

    a. 97.6°F

    b. 98.2°F

    c. 99.7°F

    d. Cannot be determined.

29. What is the device used to measure temperature called?

    a. Thermos

    b. Thermometer

    c. Thermostat

    d. Thermocouple

30. What are the two important parts of a thermometer?

    a. Temperature sensor and calibration markings

    b. Temperature sensor and scale

    c. Calibration markings and scale

    d. Bulb and scale

31. Which body part is typically used for temperature measurement by swallowing a small

thermometer?

    a. Anus

    b. Ear

    c. Mouth

    d. Gut

32. What is the typical daytime temperature reading for gut measurements in healthy adults?

    a. 97.6°F

    b. 98.2°F

    c. 99.7°F

    d. Cannot be determined.

33. Which body part is typically used for temperature measurement over the temporal artery?

    a. Anus

    b. Ear

    c. Mouth

    d. Forehead

34. What is the purpose of calibration markings on a thermometer?

    a. To indicate the type of liquid used in the thermometer.

    b. To indicate the temperature range of the thermometer

    c. To indicate the body part used for temperature measurement.

    d. To indicate the brand of the thermometer

35. Which type of thermometer uses colored alcohol instead of mercury?

    a. Oral thermometer

    b. Rectal thermometer

    c. Tympanic thermometer

    d. Alcohol thermometer

36. Which body part typically has the highest temperature reading in healthy adults?

    a. Anus

    b. Ear

    c. Mouth

    d. Vagina

37. Which body part typically has the lowest temperature reading in healthy adults?

    a.   Anus

    b.   Ear

    c.   Mouth

    d.   Under the arm

38. Which type of thermometer is commonly used in hospitals and clinics?

    a.   Liquid-filled thermometer

    b.   Digital thermometer

    c.   Infrared thermometer

    d.   Glass thermometer

39. Which type of thermometer measures temperature without contacting the body?

    a.   Liquid-filled thermometer

    b.   Digital thermometer

    c.   Infrared thermometer

    d.   Glass thermometer

40. What is the purpose of the temperature sensor in a thermometer?

    a. To convert physical change into a number

    b. To hold the liquid used in the thermometer.

    c. To indicate the temperature range of the thermometer

    d. To indicate the type of liquid used in the thermometer.

41. What is the normal body temperature range for adults?

    a. 95°F to 98°F

    b. 97°F to 99°F

    c. 98°F to 100°F

    d. 99°F to 102°F

42. What is the normal body temperature range for infants?

    a. 95°F to 98°F

    b. 97°F to 99°F

    c. 98°F to 100°F

    d. 99°F to 102°F

43. What is the term for a fever that lasts for a long period of time?

     a.   Acute fever

     b.   Chronic fever

     c.   Mild fever

     d.   Severe fever

44. What is the term for a fever that comes and goes?

     a.   Acute fever

     b.   Chronic fever

     c.   Intermittent fever

     d.   Remittent fever

45. What is the term for a fever that remains at a constant level?

     a.   Acute fever

     b.   Chronic fever

     c.   Intermittent fever

     d.   Remittent fever

46. What is the term for a fever that is caused by a bacterial infection?

  a. Viral fever

  b. Bacterial fever

  c. Fungal fever

  d. Parasitic fever

47. What is the term for a fever that is caused by a viral infection?

  a. Viral fever

  b. Bacterial fever

  c. Fungal fever

  d. Parasitic fever

48. What is the term for a fever that is caused by a fungal infection?

  a. Viral fever

  b. Bacterial fever

  c. Fungal fever

  d. Parasitic fever

49. What is the term for a fever that is caused by a parasitic infection?

   a. Viral fever

   b. Bacterial fever

   c. Fungal fever

   d. Parasitic fever

50. What is the term for a fever that is caused by an unknown source?

   a. Idiopathic fever

   b. Acute fever

   c. Chronic fever

   d. Remittent fever

51. What is the term for a fever that is caused by an allergic reaction?

   a. Allergic fever

   b. Anaphylactic fever

   c. Hypersensitivity fever

   d. Immune fever

52. What is the term for a fever that is caused by a drug reaction?

    a.   Drug fever

    b.   Allergic fever

    c.   Hypersensitivity fever

    d.   Immune fever

53. What is the term for a fever that is caused by a tumor?

    a.   Tumor fever

    b.   Cancer fever

    c.   Neoplastic fever

    d.   Malignant fever

54. What is the term for a fever that is caused by a blood clot?

    a.   Thrombotic fever

    b.   Embolic fever

    c.   Coagulation fever

    d.   Clotting fever

55. What is the term for a fever that is caused by a metabolic disorder?

     a.   Metabolic fever

     b.   Endocrine fever

     c.   Thyroid fever

     d.   Adrenal fever

56. What is the term for a fever that is caused by heat stroke?

     a.   Heat fever

     b.   Sunstroke fever

     c.   Hyperthermia fever

     d.   Heat exhaustion fever

57. What is the term for a fever that is caused by a cold exposure?

     a.   Cold fever

     b.   Hypothermia fever

     c.   Frostbite fever

     d.   Chilblain fever

58. What is the term for a fever that is caused by a central nervous system disorder?

    a.   Neurological fever

    b.   Brain fever

    c.   Encephalitis fever

    d.   Meningitis fever

59. What is the term for a fever that is caused by an autoimmune disorder?

    a.   Autoimmune fever

    b.   Inflammatory fever

    c.   Rheumatic fever

    d.   Lupus fever

60. What is the term for a fever that is caused by a psychological disorder?

    a.   Psychogenic fever

    b.   Mental fever

    c.   Emotional fever

    d.   Behavioral fever

61. Which type of thermometer is considered the most accurate liquid-filled thermometer?

    a.   Colored liquid-filled thermometer

    b.   Electronic thermometer

    c.   Mercury-in-glass thermometer

    d.   Contact thermometer.

62. Why must the tube in a mercury-in-glass thermometer be very narrow?

    a.   To make the thermometer more durable

    b.   To make the thermometer easier to read

    c.   To minimize the amount of mercury in the thermometer

    d.   To make the thermometer more accurate

63. Why is the mercury in the tube of a mercury-in-glass thermometer much less than in the bulb?

    a.   To make the thermometer more durable

    b.   To make the thermometer easier to read

    c.   To minimize the effect of temperature of the tube

    d.   To make the thermometer more accurate

64. What is the method of pushing the mercury back into the bulb from the stem called?

   a. Shaken up

   b. Shaken down

   c. Shaken left.

   d. Shaken right.

65. What is the accuracy of most electronic thermometers?

   a. 0.1°F

   b. 0.2°F

   c. 0.5°F

   d. 1°F

66. What should be done to ensure the accuracy of an electronic thermometer?

   a. Periodical recalibration

   b. Shaking it down

   c. Cleaning it with alcohol

   d. Replacing the battery

67. How do contact thermometers measure temperature?

    a. By using colored liquid

    b. By using mercury

    c. By using electronic sensors

    d. By using infrared technology

68. Which type of thermometer is not affected by the temperature of the tube?

    a. Colored liquid-filled thermometer

    b. Electronic thermometer

    c. Mercury-in-glass thermometer

    d. Contact thermometer.

69. What happens to the reading on a glass thermometer once it is removed from a patient?

    a. It decreases.

    b. It increases.

    c. It remains without change.

    d. It becomes inaccurate.

70. What must the bulb of a glass thermometer come in contact with to change the reading?

    a. Something with a lower temperature

    b. Something with a higher temperature

    c. Something with the same temperature

    d. Nothing, the reading cannot be changed.

71. Why are mercury-in-glass thermometers not commonly used anymore?

    a. They were too expensive.

    b. They are not accurate.

    c. They are difficult to read.

    d. Mercury is a toxic metal.

72. What is the advantage of colored liquid-filled thermometers over mercury-in-glass

    thermometers?

    a. They are more accurate.

    b. They are easier to read.

    c. They were less expensive.

    d. They are more durable.

73. What is the disadvantage of electronic thermometers compared to glass thermometers?

    a. They are less accurate.

    b. They were more expensive.

    c. They require calibration.

    d. They are not as durable.

74. What is the advantage of contact thermometers over glass thermometers?

    a. They are more accurate.

    b. They are easier to read.

    c. They were less expensive.

    d. They do not require shaking down.

75. What is the main disadvantage of using a glass thermometer for measuring body temperature?

    a. It is not accurate.

    b. It is difficult to read.

    c. It is fragile and can break easily.

    d. It takes a long time to get a reading.

76. What is the main advantage of using an electronic thermometer for measuring body

   temperature?

   a. It is more accurate than other types of thermometers.

   b. It is easier to read than other types of thermometers.

   c. It is less expensive than other types of thermometers.

   d. It is faster than other types of thermometers.

77. What is the main disadvantage of using a contact thermometer for measuring body

   temperature?

   a. It is less accurate than other types of thermometers.

   b. It is more expensive than other types of thermometers.

   c. It requires physical contact with the patient.

   d. It is slower than other types of thermometers.

78. What is the advantage of using a digital thermometer over a mercury-in-glass thermometer?

   a. It is more accurate.

   b. It is easier to read.

   c. It is less expensive.

   d. It is more durable.

79. What is the main disadvantage of using a glass thermometer for measuring temperature in a

laboratory setting?

    a.   It is not accurate.

    b.   It is difficult to read.

    c.   It is fragile and can break easily.

    d.   It takes a long time to get a reading.

80. What is the advantage of using a contact thermometer over an infrared thermometer?

    a.   It is more accurate.

    b.   It is easier to use.

    c.   It is less expensive.

    d.   It can measure temperature in liquids and solids.

81. What is the main disadvantage of using an infrared thermometer for measuring body

temperature?

    a.   It is less accurate than other types of thermometers.

    b.   It is more expensive than other types of thermometers.

    c.   It requires physical contact with the patient.

    d.   It can be affected by environmental factors.

82. What is the advantage of using a bimetallic thermometer over a glass thermometer?

    a. It is more accurate.

    b. It is easier to read.

    c. It is less expensive.

    d. It can measure a wider range of temperatures.

83. What is the main disadvantage of using a bimetallic thermometer?

    a. It is less accurate than other types of thermometers.

    b. It is more expensive than other types of thermometers.

    c. It requires calibration.

    d. It is slower than other types of thermometers.

84. What is the advantage of using a liquid crystal thermometer over a glass thermometer?

    a. It is more accurate.

    b. It is easier to read.

    c. It is less expensive.

    d. It can measure temperature changes over time.

85. What is the main disadvantage of using a liquid crystal thermometer?

    a. It is less accurate than other types of thermometers.

    b. It is more expensive than other types of thermometers.

    c. It requires calibration.

    d. It is affected by ambient temperature and humidity.

86. What is the advantage of using a thermocouple thermometer over other types of thermometers?

    a. It is more accurate.

    b. It is easier to read.

    c. It can measure a wider range of temperatures.

    d. It is less expensive.

87. What is the main disadvantage of using a thermocouple thermometer?

    a. It is less accurate than other types of thermometers.

    b. It is more expensive than other types of thermometers.

    c. It requires calibration.

    d. It is more difficult to use than other types of thermometers.

88. What is the advantage of using a resistance thermometer over a glass thermometer?

    a. It is more accurate.

    b. It is easier to read.

    c. It can measure a wider range of temperatures.

    d. It is less expensive.

89. What is the main disadvantage of using a resistance thermometer?

    a. It is less accurate than other types of thermometers.

    b. It is more expensive than other types of thermometers.

    c. It requires calibration.

    d. It is affected by ambient temperature and humidity.

90. What is the advantage of using a temperature data logger over other types of thermometers?

    a. It is more accurate.

    b. It can measure temperature changes over time.

    c. It is less expensive.

    d. It is easier to use.

91. What is the main disadvantage of using a temperature data logger?

    a.   It is less accurate than other types of thermometers.

    b.   It is more expensive than other types of thermometers.

    c.   It requires calibration.

    d.   It requires a computer or other device to download and analyze the data.

92. What is the advantage of using an infrared thermometer?

    a.   It is more accurate than other types of thermometers.

    b.   It can measure temperature without touching the object being measured.

    c.   It can measure a wider range of temperatures.

    d.   It is less expensive than other types of thermometers.

93. What is the main disadvantage of using an infrared thermometer?

    a.   It is less accurate than other types of thermometers.

    b.   It is more expensive than other types of thermometers.

    c.   It requires calibration.

    d.   It can only measure surface temperature, not internal temperature.

94. What is the advantage of using a bimetallic thermometer?

    a. It is more accurate than other types of thermometers.

    b. It is easier to read.

    c. It can measure a wider range of temperatures.

    d. It is less expensive than other types of thermometers.

95. What is the main disadvantage of using a bimetallic thermometer?

    a. It is less accurate than other types of thermometers.

    b. It is more expensive than other types of thermometers.

    c. It requires calibration.

    d. It can only measure a limited range of temperatures.

96. What is the advantage of using a thermocouple thermometer?

    a. It is more accurate than other types of thermometers.

    b. It can measure temperature without touching the object being measured.

    c. It can measure a wider range of temperatures.

    d. It is less expensive than other types of thermometers.

97. What is the main disadvantage of using a thermocouple thermometer?

    a. It is less accurate than other types of thermometers.

    b. It is more expensive than other types of thermometers.

    c. It requires calibration.

    d. It is more fragile than other types of thermometers.

98. What is the advantage of using a resistance thermometer?

    a. It is more accurate than other types of thermometers.

    b. It can measure temperature without touching the object being measured.

    c. It can measure a wider range of temperatures.

    d. It is less expensive than other types of thermometers.

99. What is the main disadvantage of using a resistance thermometer?

    a. It is more expensive than other types of thermometers.

    b. It requires calibration.

    c. It can only measure a limited range of temperatures.

    d. It is more fragile than other types of thermometers.

100.What is the advantage of using a liquid-in-glass thermometer?

    a. It is more accurate than other types of thermometers.

    b. It is easier to read.

    c. It can measure a wider range of temperatures.

    d. It is less expensive than other types of thermometers

PART-SEVEN
ANSWER TO MEDICAL ASSISTANT QUESTIONS

1. Answer: B

   Increase

2. Answer: A

   Decrease

3. Answer: C

   Increase during the night and decrease during the day.

4. Answer: B

   Increase

5. Answer: B

   Children

6. Answer: B

   Increase

7. Answer: B

   Decrease throughout the night.

8. Answer: A

   Increase at night.

9. Answer: B

Decrease at night.

10. Answer: D

All of the above

11. Answer: B

Decrease - Poor sleep quality or insomnia can cause a decrease in body temperature as the body is not

able to regulate its temperature properly.

12. Answer: D

Cannot be determined - The effect of changes to shift work on body temperature can vary depending.

on the individual and the specific shift schedule.

13. Answer: C

No effect - Waking up at unusual times typically does not have a significant effect on the body.

temperature.

14. Answer: D

Cannot be determined - The effect of jet lag on body temperature can vary depending on the

individual and the specific travel schedule.

15. Answer: B

Decrease - Body temperature generally decreases at night as the body prepares for sleep.

16. Answer: B

    Increase - Sustained physical activity can cause an increase in body temperature as the body produces.

    more heat.

17. Answer: B

    Increase - Sustained physical activity can cause an increase in body temperature in children as well as

    adults.

18. Answer: B

    Increase - Emotional or mental stress can cause an increase in body temperature as the body produces.

    more heat.

19. Answer: A

    Increase at night - Short-term sleep deprivation can cause an increase in body temperature at night as

    the body tries to regulate its temperature.

20. Answer: B

    Decrease at night - Long-term sleep deprivation can cause a decrease in body temperature at night as

    the body is not able to regulate its temperature properly.

21. Answer: C

    Mouth

22. Answer: A

    Anus

23. Answer: B

    Ear

24. Answer: D

    Under the arm

25. Answer: D

    Vagina

26. Answer: C

    99.7°F

27. Answer: B

    98.2°F

28. Answer: A

    97.6°F

29. Answer: B

    Thermometer

30. Answer: A

    Temperature sensor and calibration markings

31. Answer D

    Gut: The part of the body typically used for temperature measurement by swallowing a small

    thermometer.

32. Answer B

98.2°F: The typical daytime temperature reading for gut measurements in healthy adults.

33. Answer D

Forehead: The body part typically used for temperature measurement over the temporal artery.

34. Answer B

To indicate the temperature range of the thermometer: The purpose of calibration markings on a thermometer.

35. Answer D

Alcohol thermometer: The type of thermometer that uses colored alcohol instead of mercury.

36. Answer A

Anus: The body part that typically has the highest temperature reading in healthy adults.

37. Answer D

Under the arm: The body part that typically has the lowest temperature reading in healthy adults.

38. Answer B

Digital thermometer: The type of thermometer commonly used in hospitals and clinics.

39. Answer C

Infrared thermometer: The type of thermometer that measures temperature without making contact with the body.

40. Answer A

To convert physical change into a number: The purpose of the temperature sensor in a thermometer.

41. Answer B

97°F to 99°F: The normal body temperature range for adults.

42. Answer C

98°F to 100°F: The normal body temperature range for infants.

43. Answer B

Chronic fever: The term for a fever that lasts for a long period of time.

44. Answer C

Intermittent fever: The term for a fever that comes and goes.

45. Answer D

Remittent fever: The term for a fever that remains at a constant level.

46. Answer B

Bacterial fever: The term for a fever that is caused by a bacterial infection.

47. Answer A

Viral fever: The term for a fever that is caused by a viral infection.

48. Answer C

Fungal fever: The term for a fever that is caused by a fungal infection.

49. Answer D

Parasitic fever: The term for a fever that is caused by a parasitic infection.

50. Answer A

Idiopathic fever: The term for a fever that is caused by an unknown source.

51. Answer C

Hypersensitivity fever: The term for a fever that is caused by an allergic reaction.

52. Answer A

Drug fever: The term for a fever that is caused by a drug reaction.

53. Answer C

Neoplastic fever: The term for a fever that is caused by a tumor.

54. Answer B

Embolic fever: The term for a fever that is caused by a blood clot.

55. Answer B

Endocrine fever: The term for a fever that is caused by a metabolic disorder.

56. Answer C

Hyperthermia fever: The term for a fever that is caused by a heat stroke.

57. Answer B

Hypothermia fever: The term for a fever that is caused by a cold exposure.

58. Answer A

Neurological fever: The term for a fever that is caused by a central nervous system disorder.

59. Answer B

Inflammatory fever: The term for a fever that is caused by an autoimmune disorder.

60. Answer A

Psychogenic fever: The term for a fever that is caused by a psychological disorder.

61. Answer: C

Mercury-in-glass thermometer

62. Answer: C

To minimize the amount of mercury in the thermometer

63. Answer: C

To minimize the effect of temperature of the tube

64. Answer: B

Shaken down

65. Answer: B

0.2°F

66. Answer: A

Periodical recalibration

67. Answer: C

   By using electronic sensors

68. Answer: B

   Electronic thermometer

69. Answer: C

   It remains without change

70. Answer: B

   Something with a higher temperature

71. Answer: D

   Mercury is a toxic metal.

72. Answer: B

   They are easier to read.

73. Answer: C

   They require calibration.

74. Answer: D

   They do not require shaking down.

75. Answer: C

   It is fragile and can break easily.

76. Answer: D

It is faster than other types of thermometers.

77. Answer: C

It requires physical contact with the patient.

78. Answer: B

It is easier to read.

79. Answer: C

It is fragile and can break easily.

80. Answer: D

It can measure temperature in liquids and solids.

81. Answer D

It can be affected by environmental factors.

82. Answer: D

It can measure a wider range of temperatures.

83. Answer: A

It is less accurate than other types of thermometers.

84. Answer: D

It can measure temperature changes over time.

85. Answer: D

It is affected by ambient temperature and humidity.

86. Answer: C

It can measure a wider range of temperatures.

87. Answer: C

It requires calibration.

88. Answer: A

It is more accurate.

89. Answer: D

It is affected by ambient temperature and humidity.

90. Answer: B

It can measure temperature changes over time.

91. Answer: D

It requires a computer or other device to download and analyze the data.

92. Answer: B

It can measure temperature without touching the object being measured.

93. Answer: D

It can only measure surface temperature, not internal temperature

94. Answer: B

It is easier to read.

95. Answer: D

It can only measure a limited range of temperatures.

96. Answer: C

It can measure a wider range of temperatures.

97. Answer: A

It is less accurate than other types of thermometers.

98. Answer: A

It is more accurate than other types of thermometers.

99. Answer: C

It can only measure a limited range of temperatures.

100.Answer: B

It is easier to read.

MEDICAL ASSISTANT CERTIFICATION
EXAMINATION STUDY GUIDE
PART-EIGHT

1. What is blood pressure?

    a. The pressure exerted by circulating blood upon the walls of blood vessels.

    b. The pressure exerted by the heart upon the walls of blood vessels.

    c. The pressure exerted by the lungs upon the walls of blood vessels.

    d. The pressure exerted by the kidneys upon the walls of blood vessels.

2. What is the difference between systolic and diastolic blood pressure?

    a. Systolic is the maximum pressure during contraction, while diastolic is the minimum pressure during relaxation.

    b. Systolic is the minimum pressure during relaxation, while diastolic is the maximum pressure during contraction.

    c. Systolic and diastolic are the same thing.

    d. Systolic and diastolic are unrelated to blood pressure.

3. What is the usual location for measuring blood pressure?

    a. The inside of the wrist

    b. The inside of the elbow

    c. The back of the hand

    d. The back of the knee

4. What is the typical blood pressure reading for a healthy adult?

    a. 80/60 mmHg

    b. 120/80 mmHg

    c. 160/100 mmHg

    d. 200/120 mmHg

5. What causes blood pressure to decrease as blood moves away from the heart?

    a. Resistance to flow in blood vessels

    b. Gravity

    c. Valves in veins

    d. Pumping from contracting skeletal muscles

6. Which part of the heart is responsible for the systolic blood pressure reading?

    a. The left atrium

    b. The right atrium

    c. The left ventricle

    d. The right ventricle

7. Which part of the heart is responsible for the diastolic blood pressure reading?

    a. The left atrium

    b. The right atrium

    c. The left ventricle

    d. The right ventricle

8. What is the role of valves in veins in relation to blood pressure?

   a. They help to pump blood through the veins.

   b. They prevent blood from flowing backwards in the veins.

   c. They regulate the amount of blood flowing through the veins.

   d. They have no effect on blood pressure.

9. Which blood vessels experience the most rapid drop in blood pressure?

   a. Arteries

   b. Veins

   c. Capillaries

   d. Arterioles

10. What is the unit of measurement for blood pressure?

    a. Liters per minute

    b. Millimeters of mercury (mmHg)

    c. Beats per minute.

    d. Pascals (Pa)

11. What is the name of the artery usually used to measure blood pressure?

    a. Radial artery

    b. Carotid artery

    c. Brachial artery

    d. Femoral artery

12. What is the normal range for diastolic blood pressure?

    a. 60-80 mmHg

    b. 80-100 mmHg

    c. 100-120 mmHg

    d. 120-140 mmHg

13. What is the normal range for systolic blood pressure?

    a. 90-120 mmHg

    b. 120-140 mmHg

    c. 140-160 mmHg

    d. 160-180 mmHg

14. What is the name for the resistance to flow in blood vessels that causes blood pressure to decrease as blood moves away from the heart?

    a. Vascular resistance

    b. Cardiac resistance

    c. Pulmonary resistance

    d. Renal resistance

15. Which of the following can influence blood pressure at different places in the body?

    a. Valves in veins

    b. Gravity

    c. Pumping from contracting skeletal muscles

    d. All of the above

16. What is the name for the maximum arterial pressure during contraction of the left ventricle of the heart?

    a. Systolic blood pressure

    b. Diastolic blood pressure

    c. Mean arterial pressure.

    d. Pulse pressure

17. What is the name for the minimum arterial pressure during relaxation of the heart?

    a. Systolic blood pressure

    b. Diastolic blood pressure

    c. Mean arterial pressure.

    d. Pulse pressure

18. What is the name for the average pressure in the arteries during one cardiac cycle?

    a. Systolic blood pressure

    b. Diastolic blood pressure

    c. Mean arterial pressure.

    d. Pulse pressure

19. What is the name for the difference between systolic and diastolic blood pressure?

    a. Systolic pressure

    b. Diastolic pressure

    c. Mean arterial pressure.

    d. Pulse pressure

20. What is the name for the pressure exerted by the heart upon the walls of blood vessels?

    a. Blood pressure

    b. Cardiac pressure

    c. Vascular pressure

    d. Pulmonary pressure

21. What is the medical term for low blood pressure?

    a. Hypertension

    b. Hypotension

    c. Hyperglycemia

    d. Hypoglycemia

22. What is the most common symptom of low blood pressure?

    a. Headache

    b. Nausea

    c. Dizziness

    d. Chest pain

23. What is the term for low blood pressure that occurs when a person changes position from sitting or lying to standing?

    a. Orthostatic hypotension

    b. Postural hypotension

    c. Systolic hypotension

    d. Diastolic hypotension

24. What is the most severe form of low blood pressure?

    a. Hypertension

    b. Orthostatic hypotension

    c. Shock

    d. Bradycardia

25. What type of testing can be done to determine the cause of low blood pressure?

    a. Blood test

    b. Cardiac testing

    c. Radiologic studies

    d. All of the above

26. What is a common cause of low blood pressure in pregnant women?

    a. Heart problems

    b. Dehydration

    c. Blood loss

    d. Circulatory system expansion

27. What type of heart problem can cause low blood pressure?

    a. High heart rate

    b. Low heart rate

    c. Enlarged heart.

    d. Blocked arteries

28. What is the term for low blood pressure caused by a heart attack?

   a. Cardiogenic shock

   b. Hypovolemic shock

   c. Anaphylactic shock

   d. Septic shock

29. What is the term for low blood pressure caused by kidney failure?

   a. Cardiogenic shock

   b. Hypovolemic shock

   c. Anaphylactic shock

   d. Septic shock

30. What is the treatment for low blood pressure determined by?

   a. The severity of symptoms

   b. The cause of low blood pressure

   c. The age of the patient

   d. The patient's weight.

31. What is the normal range for blood pressure?

   a. 80/60 mmHg

   b. 120/80 mmHg

   c. 140/90 mmHg

   d. 160/100 mmHg

32. What is the term for low blood pressure that occurs during exercise?

  a. Exercise-induced hypotension

  b. Postural hypotension

  c. Systolic hypotension

  d. Diastolic hypotension

33. What is the term for low blood pressure caused by dehydration?

  a. Hypovolemic shock

  b. Cardiogenic shock

  c. Anaphylactic shock

  d. Septic shock

34. What is the term for low blood pressure caused by an allergic reaction?

  a. Anaphylactic shock

  b. Hypovolemic shock

  c. Cardiogenic shock

  d. Septic shock

35. What is the term for low blood pressure caused by blood loss?

  a. Hypovolemic shock

  b. Cardiogenic shock

  c. Anaphylactic shock

  d. Septic shock

36. What is the term for low blood pressure caused by an infection?

    a. Septic shock

    b. Hypovolemic shock

    c. Cardiogenic shock

    d. Anaphylactic shock

37. What is the term for low blood pressure caused by a medication?

    a. Drug-induced hypotension

    b. Postural hypotension

    c. Systolic hypotension

    d. Diastolic hypotension

38. What is the term for low blood pressure caused by a nerve disorder?

    a. Neurogenic hypotension

    b. Postural hypotension

    c. Systolic hypotension

    d. Diastolic hypotension

39. What is the term for low blood pressure caused by a hormonal imbalance?

    a. Endocrine hypotension

    b. Postural hypotension

    c. Systolic hypotension

    d. Diastolic hypotension

40. What is the term for low blood pressure caused by a blood clot?

   a. Pulmonary embolism

   b. Deep vein thrombosis

   c. Atherosclerosis

   d. Coronary artery disease

41. What is the term for low blood pressure caused by a heart condition?

   a. Cardiogenic shock

   b. Hypovolemic shock

   c. Anaphylactic shock

   d. Septic shock

42. What is the term for low blood pressure caused by a spinal cord injury?

   a. Neurogenic shock

   b. Hypovolemic shock

   c. Anaphylactic shock

   d. Septic shock

43. What is the term for low blood pressure caused by a brain injury?

   a. Neurogenic shock

   b. Hypovolemic shock

   c. Anaphylactic shock

   d. Septic shock

44. What is the term for low blood pressure caused by a severe allergic reaction?

   a. Anaphylactic shock

   b. Hypovolemic shock

   c. Cardiogenic shock

   d. Septic shock

45. What is the term for low blood pressure caused by a blood infection?

   a. Septic shock

   b. Hypovolemic shock

   c. Cardiogenic shock

   d. Anaphylactic shock

46. What is the term for low blood pressure caused by a malfunctioning adrenal gland?

   a. Adrenal insufficiency

   b. Hypovolemic shock

   c. Cardiogenic shock

   d. Anaphylactic shock

47. What is the term for low blood pressure caused by a blood clot in the lungs?

   a. Pulmonary embolism

   b. Deep vein thrombosis

   c. Atherosclerosis

   d. Coronary artery disease

48. What is the term for low blood pressure caused by a bacterial infection in the bloodstream?

    a. Septic shock

    b. Hypovolemic shock

    c. Cardiogenic shock

    d. Anaphylactic shock

49. What is the term for low blood pressure caused by a severe burn injury?

    a. Burn shock.

    b. Hypovolemic shock

    c. Cardiogenic shock

    d. Anaphylactic shock

50. What is the term for low blood pressure caused by a reaction to anesthesia?

    a. Anesthetic-induced hypotension

    b. Postural hypotension

    c. Systolic hypotension

    d. Diastolic hypotension

51. What can cause a life-threatening drop in blood pressure due to a severe infection in the body?

    a. Hypothyroidism

    b. Hyperthyroidism

    c. Septicemia

    d. Anaphylaxis

52. What condition can cause low blood pressure due to a lack of red blood cells?

    a. Hypothyroidism

    b. Hyperthyroidism

    c. Anemia

    d. Septicemia

53. What can cause low blood pressure due to a severe allergic reaction?

    a. Hypothyroidism

    b. Hyperthyroidism

    c. Anemia

    d. Anaphylaxis

54. What can cause low blood pressure due to a lack of nutrients such as vitamins B-12 and folate?

    a. Hypothyroidism

    b. Hyperthyroidism

    c. Anemia

    d. Septicemia

55. What can cause low blood pressure due to adrenal insufficiency?

    a. Hypothyroidism

    b. Hyperthyroidism

    c. Anemia

    d. Addison's disease

56. What can cause low blood pressure due to hypoglycemia?

    a. Hypothyroidism

    b. Hyperthyroidism

    c. Anemia

    d. Low blood sugar

57. What can cause low blood pressure due to internal bleeding or major injury?

    a. Hypothyroidism

    b. Hyperthyroidism

    c. Anemia

    d. High blood loss

58. What can cause low blood pressure due to overactive thyroid?

    a. Hypothyroidism

    b. Hyperthyroidism

    c. Anemia

    d. Addison's disease

59. What can cause low blood pressure due to underactive thyroid?

    a. Hypothyroidism

    b. Hyperthyroidism

    c. Anemia

    d. Septicemia

60. What can cause low blood pressure due to insect venom or certain medications?

    a. Hypothyroidism

    b. Hyperthyroidism

    c. Anemia

    d. Anaphylaxis

61. What can cause low blood pressure due to dehydration?

    a. Hypothyroidism

    b. Hyperthyroidism

    c. Anemia

    d. Loss of fluids

62. What can cause low blood pressure due to heart problems?

    a. Hypothyroidism

    b. Hyperthyroidism

    c. Anemia

    d. Heart failure

63. What can cause low blood pressure due to medication side effects?

    a. Hypothyroidism

    b. Hyperthyroidism

    c. Anemia

    d. Blood pressure medication

64. What can cause low blood pressure due to nerve damage?

   a. Hypothyroidism

   b. Hyperthyroidism

   c. Anemia

   d. Autonomic neuropathy

65. What can cause low blood pressure due to pregnancy?

   a. Hypothyroidism

   b. Hyperthyroidism

   c. Anemia

   d. Pregnancy-induced hypertension

66. What can cause low blood pressure due to a heart attack?

   a. Hypothyroidism

   b. Hyperthyroidism

   c. Anemia

   d. Myocardial infarction

67. What can cause low blood pressure due to a blood clot?

   a. Hypothyroidism

   b. Hyperthyroidism

   c. Anemia

   d. Deep vein thrombosis

68. What can cause low blood pressure due to a reaction to anesthesia?

    a. Hypothyroidism

    b. Hyperthyroidism

    c. Anemia

    d. Anesthesia-induced hypotension

69. What can cause low blood pressure due to a sudden change in position?

    a. Hypothyroidism

    b. Hyperthyroidism

    c. Anemia

    d. Orthostatic hypotension

70. What can cause low blood pressure due to excessive alcohol consumption?

    a. Hypothyroidism

    b. Hyperthyroidism

    c. Anemia

    d. Alcohol-induced hypotension

71. What is postural/ orthostatic hypotension?

    a. A sudden drop in blood pressure after eating.

    b. A sudden drop in blood pressure when standing up from a sitting or lying position.

    c. A sudden drop in blood pressure due to medication side effects

    d. A sudden drop in blood pressure due to heart problems

72. What are some symptoms of postural/ orthostatic hypotension?

    a. Nausea and vomiting

    b. Chest pain and shortness of breath

    c. Dizziness and feeling lightheaded.

    d. Headache and confusion

73. What are some causes of postural/ orthostatic hypotension?

    a. High blood pressure and heart disease

    b. Dehydration and prolonged bed rest

    c. Diabetes and burns.

    d. All of the above

74. What medications can cause postural/ orthostatic hypotension?

    a. Antidepressants and drugs to treat high blood pressure.

    b. Medications for erectile dysfunction

    c. Medications for Parkinson's disease

    d. All of the above

75. What is postprandial hypotension?

    a. A sudden drop in blood pressure after eating.

    b. A sudden drop in blood pressure when standing up from a sitting or lying position.

    c. A sudden drop in blood pressure due to medication side effects

    d. A sudden drop in blood pressure due to heart problems

76. Who is most likely to be affected by postprandial hypotension?

    a. People with low blood pressure

    b. People with high blood pressure

    c. People with heart disease

    d. People with autonomic nervous system disorders

77. What are some ways to reduce symptoms of postprandial hypotension?

    a. Eat smaller portions and low carbohydrate meals.

    b. Increase salt intake.

    c. Increase fluid intake.

    d. All of the above

78. What is neutrally mediated hypotension?

    a. A sudden drop in blood pressure after eating.

    b. A sudden drop in blood pressure when standing up from a sitting or lying position.

    c. A sudden drop in blood pressure due to medication side effects

    d. A sudden drop in blood pressure due to miscommunication between heart and brain

79. Who is most likely to be affected by neutrally mediated hypotension?

    a. Older adults

    b. Young people

    c. People with heart disease

    d. People with autonomic nervous system disorders

80. What are some symptoms of neutrally mediated hypotension?

   a. Dizziness and feeling lightheaded.

   b. Nausea and vomiting

   c. Fainting

   d. All of the above

81. What is the cause of neutrally mediated hypotension?

   a. Dehydration

   b. Heart problems

   c. Miscommunication between heart and brain

   d. Medication side effects

82. What are some neurological disorders that can cause postural/ orthostatic hypotension?

   a. Parkinson's disease

   b. Multiple sclerosis

   c. Guillain-Barre syndrome

   d. All of the above

83. What is the treatment for postural/ orthostatic hypotension?

   a. Increasing salt intake

   b. Drinking more fluids

   c. Wearing compression stockings

   d. All of the above

84. What is the treatment for neutrally mediated hypotension?

    a. Medications to increase blood pressure.

    b. Drinking more fluids

    c. Avoiding triggers that cause symptoms.

    d. All of the above

85. What is the difference between low blood pressure and hypotension?

    a. There is no difference, they mean the same thing.

    b. Low blood pressure is a normal variation, while hypotension is a medical condition.

    c. Low blood pressure is a medical condition, while hypotension is a normal variation.

    d. Low blood pressure and hypotension are both medical conditions.

86. What is the difference between postural/ orthostatic hypotension and neutrally mediated hypotension?

    a. Postural/ orthostatic hypotension is caused by dehydration, while neutrally mediated hypotension is caused by miscommunication between heart and brain.

    b. Postural/ orthostatic hypotension mostly affects young people, while neutrally mediated hypotension mostly affects older people.

    c. Postural/ orthostatic hypotension is a sudden drop in blood pressure when standing up, while neutrally mediated hypotension is a sudden drop in blood pressure due to miscommunication between heart and brain.

    d. Postural/ orthostatic hypotension is a normal variation, while neutrally mediated hypotension is a medical condition.

87. What is the difference between postprandial hypotension and postural/ orthostatic hypotension?

   a. Postprandial hypotension is a sudden drop in blood pressure when standing up, while postural/ orthostatic hypotension is a sudden drop in blood pressure after eating.

   b. Postprandial hypotension mostly affects young people, while postural/ orthostatic hypotension mostly affects older people.

   c. Postprandial hypotension is a normal variation, while postural/ orthostatic hypotension is a medical condition.

   d. Postprandial hypotension is a sudden drop in blood pressure after eating, while postural/ orthostatic hypotension is a sudden drop in blood pressure when standing up from a sitting or lying position.

88. What is the difference between low blood pressure and high blood pressure?

   a. Low blood pressure is a normal variation, while high blood pressure is a medical condition.

   b. Low blood pressure is a medical condition, while high blood pressure is a normal variation.

   c. Low blood pressure and high blood pressure are both normal variations.

   d. Low blood pressure and high blood pressure are both medical conditions.

89. What is the difference between hypotension and hypertension?

   a. Hypotension is a normal variation, while hypertension is a medical condition.

   b. Hypotension is a medical condition, while hypertension is a normal variation.

   c. Hypotension and hypertension are both normal variations.

   d. Hypotension and hypertension are both medical conditions.

90. What are some lifestyle changes that can help manage low blood pressure?

   a.   Drinking more fluids

   b.   Eating smaller, more frequent meals

   c.   Avoiding alcohol and caffeine

   d.   All of the above

91. What is Shy-Drager Syndrome?

   a.   A common disorder that affects the autonomic nervous system

   b.   A rare disorder that affects the voluntary nervous system

   c.   A common disorder that causes high blood pressure

   d.   A rare disorder that causes low blood pressure

92. What is the main characteristic of Shy-Drager Syndrome?

   a.   Muscle tremors

   b.   Slow movement.

   c.   Problems with coordination and speech

   d.   Severe orthostatic hypotension in combination with very high blood pressure when lying down.

93. What does the autonomic nervous system control?

   a.   Voluntary functions such as blood pressure, heart rate, breathing and digestion.

   b.   Involuntary functions such as blood pressure, heart rate, breathing and digestion.

   c.   Voluntary functions such as movement and speech

   d.   Involuntary functions such as movement and speech

94. What is orthostatic hypotension?

    a. A sudden drop in blood pressure when standing up.

    b. A sudden increase in blood pressure when lying down.

    c. A sudden drop in blood pressure after eating.

    d. A sudden increase in blood pressure after eating.

95. What is the risk factor for low blood pressure on standing after eating?

    a. Age

    b. Medications

    c. Certain diseases

    d. All of the above

96. What medication has a greater risk of low blood pressure?

    a. High blood pressure medications (alpha blockers)

    b. Antibiotics

    c. Painkillers

    d. Antidepressants

97. What disease can put a person at greater risk of developing hypotension?

    a. Diabetes

    b. Cancer

    c. Asthma

    d. Allergies

98. What is incontinence?

    a. A sudden drop in blood pressure when standing up.

    b. A sudden increase in blood pressure when lying down.

    c. Loss of bladder or bowel control

    d. Loss of muscle coordination

99. What is Parkinson's disease?

    a. A common disorder that affects the autonomic nervous system

    b. A rare disorder that affects the voluntary nervous system

    c. A common disorder that causes high blood pressure

    d. A rare disorder that causes low blood pressure

100. What is the treatment for Shy-Drager Syndrome?

    a. There is no cure for Shy-Drager Syndrome

    b. Medications to manage symptoms.

    c. Surgery to repair the autonomic nervous system.

    d. All of the above

PART-EIGHT

ANSWER TO MEDICAL ASSISTANT QUESTIONS

1. Answer C

   A The pressure exerted by circulating blood upon the walls of blood vessels.

2. Answer A

   Systolic is the maximum pressure during contraction, while diastolic is the minimum

   pressure during relaxation

3. Answer B

   The inside of the elbow

4. Answer B

   120/80 mmHg

5. Answer A

   Resistance to flow in blood vessels

6. Answer C

   The left ventricle

7. Answer C

   The left ventricle

8. Answer B

   They prevent blood from flowing backwards in the veins.

9. Answer D

   Arterioles

10. Answer B

    Millimeters of mercury (mmHg)

11. Answer C

    Brachial artery

12. Answer A

    60-80   mHg

13. Answer B

    120-140 Hg

14. Answer A

    Vascular resistance

15. Answer D

    All of the above

16. Answer A

    Systolic blood pressure

17. Answer B

    Diastolic blood pressure

18. Answer C

Mean arterial pressure.

19. Answer D

Pulse pressure

20. Answer B

Cardiac pressure

21. Answer: B

Hypotension is a medical term used to describe low blood pressure, which can cause symptoms such

as dizziness, lightheadedness, and fainting.

22. Answer: C

Dizziness is a common symptom of low blood pressure, which can occur when the blood flow to

the brain is reduced.

23. Answer: A

Orthostatic hypotension is a type of low blood pressure that occurs when a person changes position

from sitting or lying to standing, which can cause dizziness, lightheadedness, and fainting.

24. Answer: C

Shock is the most severe form of low blood pressure, which can occur when the blood flow to the

organs are severely reduced, leading to organ failure.

25. Answer: D

All of the above

26. Answer: D

During pregnancy, a woman's circulatory system expands rapidly, which can cause blood pressure to

drop rapidly.

27. Answer: B

Low heart rate Bradycardia, or an extremely low heart rate, can cause low blood pressure by

preventing the body from circulating enough blood.

28. Answer: A

Cardiogenic shock is a type of shock caused by a heart attack, which can lead to low blood pressure.

pressure and organ failure.

29. Answer: B

Hypovolemic shock is a type of shock caused by kidney failure, which can lead to low blood pressure.

pressure and organ failure.

30. Answer: B

The cause of low blood pressure

The treatment for low blood pressure is determined by the underlying cause, which can

include medications, lifestyle changes, or surgery.

31. Answer: B

    120/80 mmHg the normal range for blood pressure is typically considered to be around

    120/80 mmHg, although this can vary depending on age, health status, and other factors.

32. Answer: A

    Exercise-induced hypotension is a type of low blood pressure that can occur during or after

    exercise, which can cause symptoms such as dizziness, lightheadedness, and fainting.

33. Answer: A

    Hypovolemic shock is a type of shock caused by dehydration, which can lead to low blood

    pressure and organ failure.

34. Answer: A

    Anaphylactic shock is a type of shock caused by an allergic reaction, which can lead to low

    blood pressure and organ failure.

35. Answer: A

    Hypovolemic shock is a type of shock caused by blood loss, which can lead to low blood

    pressure and organ failure.

36. Answer: A

    Septic shock is a type of shock caused by an infection, which can lead to low blood pressure

    and organ failure.

37. Answer: A

   Drug-induced hypotension is a type of low blood pressure caused by certain medications, which can cause symptoms such as dizziness, lightheadedness, and fainting.

38. Answer: A

   Neurogenic hypotension is a type of low blood pressure caused by a nerve disorder, which can cause symptoms such as dizziness, lightheadedness, and fainting.

39. Answer: A

   Endocrine hypotension is a type of low blood pressure caused by a hormonal imbalance, which can cause symptoms such as dizziness, lightheadedness, and fainting.

40. Answer: A

   Pulmonary embolism is a type of blood clot that can cause low blood pressure and other symptoms such as shortness of breath and chest pain.

41. Answer: A

   Cardiogenic shock is a type of shock caused by a heart condition, which can lead to low blood pressure and organ failure.

42. Answer: A

   Neurogenic shock is a type of shock caused by a spinal cord injury, which can lead to low blood pressure and organ failure.

43. Answer: A

   Neurogenic shock is a type of shock caused by a brain injury, which can lead to low blood

   pressure and organ failure.

44. Answer: A

   Anaphylactic shock is a type of shock caused by a severe allergic reaction, which can lead to

   low blood pressure and organ failure.

45. Answer: A

   Septic shock is a type of shock caused by a blood infection, which can lead to low blood

   pressure and organ failure.

46. Answer: A

   Adrenal insufficiency is a condition where the adrenal gland does not produce enough

   hormones, which can lead to low blood pressure and other symptoms.

47. Answer: A

   Pulmonary embolism is a type of blood clot that can cause low blood pressure and other

   symptoms such as shortness of breath and chest pain.

48. Answer: A

   Septic shock is a type of shock caused by a bacterial infection in the bloodstream, which can

   lead to low blood pressure and organ failure.

49. Answer: A

Burn shock is a type of shock caused by a severe burn injury, which can lead to low blood

pressure and organ failure.

50. Answer: A

Anesthetic-induced hypotension is a type of low blood pressure caused by a reaction to

anesthesia, which can cause symptoms such as dizziness, lightheadedness, and fainting.

51. Answer: C

Septicemia is a condition where an infection in the body enters the bloodstream, which can

lead to a life-threatening drop in blood pressure known as septic shock.

52. Answer: C

Anemia is a condition where the body doesn't produce enough red blood cells, which can

lead to low blood pressure.

53. Answer: D

Anaphylaxis is a severe and potentially life-threatening allergic reaction that can cause a drop

in blood pressure.

54. Answer: C

Anemia: A lack of nutrients such as vitamins B-12 and folate can cause anemia, which can

lead to low blood pressure.

55. Answer: D

   Adrenal insufficiency, also known as Addison's disease, is a condition where the adrenal

   gland does not produce enough hormones, which can lead to low blood pressure and other

   symptoms.

56. Answer: D

   Low blood sugar Hypoglycemia, also known as low blood sugar, can cause low blood

   pressure and other symptoms such as dizziness and confusion.

57. Answer: D

   High blood loss caused by a major injury or internal bleeding can lead to a drastic drop in

   blood pressure.

58. Answer: B

   Hyperthyroidism, or an overactive thyroid, can cause low blood pressure and other

   symptoms such as rapid heartbeat and weight loss.

59. Answer: A

   Hypothyroidism, or an underactive thyroid, can cause low blood pressure and other

   symptoms such as fatigue and weight gain.

60. Answer: D

   Anaphylaxis: Insect venom or certain medications can trigger anaphylaxis, a severe and

   potentially life-threatening allergic reaction that can cause a drop in blood pressure.

61. Answer: D.

Dehydration, or loss of fluids, can cause low blood pressure due to a decrease in blood.

Volume.

62. Answer: D

Heart failure, or a weakened heart muscle, can cause low blood pressure due to the heart's inability to pump blood effectively.

63. Answer: D

Blood pressure medication Certain medications, such as blood pressure medication, can

cause low blood pressure as a side effect.

64. Answer: D

Autonomic neuropathy, or nerve damage that affects the autonomic nervous system, can

cause low blood pressure and other symptoms.

65. Answer: D

Pregnancy-induced hypertension, or high blood pressure during pregnancy, can cause low

blood pressure as a result of treatment or other factors.

66. Answer: D

A heart attack, or myocardial infarction, can cause low blood pressure due to damage to the

heart muscle.

67. Answer: D

Deep vein thrombosis, or a blood clot in a deep vein, can cause low blood pressure as a result of decreased blood flow.

68. Answer: D

Anesthesia-induced hypotension, or low blood pressure caused by anesthesia, can occur

during surgery or other medical procedures.

69. Answer: D

Orthostatic hypotension, or low blood pressure caused by a sudden change in position, can

occur when standing up too quickly or after prolonged sitting.

70. Answer: D

Alcohol-induced hypotension, or low blood pressure caused by excessive alcohol

consumption, can occur as a result of the depressant effects of alcohol on the nervous

system.

71. Answer: B

A sudden drop in blood pressure when standing up from a sitting or lying position Postural/

orthostatic hypotension is a sudden drop in blood pressure when standing up from a sitting

or lying position, leading to symptoms of dizziness, feeling lightheaded, blurred vision, and

even fainting.

72. Answer: C

Symptoms of postural/ orthostatic hypotension include dizziness, feeling lightheaded,

blurred vision, and even fainting.

73. Answer: B

Dehydration and prolonged bed rest Causes of postural/ orthostatic hypotension include

dehydration, prolonged bed rest, diabetes, heart problems, burns, excessive heat, large

varicose veins, and certain types of neurological disorders.

74. Answer: D

All of the above

75. Answer: A

A sudden drop in blood pressure after eating. Postprandial hypotension is a sudden drop in blood

pressure after eating.

76. Answer: D

People with autonomic nervous system disorders. Postprandial hypotension is most likely to affect

people with high blood pressure or people. Suffering from autonomic nervous system disorders.

77. Answer: A

To help reduce the symptoms of postprandial hypotension, a person could eat smaller.

portions, low carbohydrate meals, or lower the dose of blood pressure medications.

78. Answer: D

A sudden drop in blood pressure due to miscommunication between heart and brain Neutrally

Mediated hypotension is a sudden drop in blood pressure due to miscommunication between the heart.

and brain.

79. Answer: B

Young people Neutrally mediated hypotension mostly affects young people.

80. Answer: D

All of the above

81. Answer C

Miscommunication between heart and brain

82. Answer D

All of the above

83. Answer D

All of the above

84. Answer C

Avoiding triggers that cause symptoms.

85. Answer B

Low blood pressure is a normal variation, while hypotension is a medical condition.

86. Answer C

Postural/ orthostatic hypotension is a sudden drop in blood pressure when standing up,

while neutrally mediated hypotension is a sudden drop in blood pressure due to

miscommunication between heart and brain

87. Answer D

Postprandial hypotension is a sudden drop in blood pressure after eating, while postural/

orthostatic hypotension is a sudden drop in blood pressure when standing up from a sitting.

or lying position

88. Answer D

Low blood pressure and high blood pressure are both medical conditions.

89. Answer D

Hypotension and hypertension are both medical conditions.

90. Answer D

All of the above

91. Answer B

A rare disorder that affects the voluntary nervous system

92. Answer D

Severe orthostatic hypotension in combination with very high blood pressure when

93. Answer B

Involuntary functions such as blood pressure, heart bate, breathing and digestion.

94. Answer A

A sudden drop in blood pressure when standing up.

95. Answer A

Age

96. Answer A

High blood pressure medications (alpha blockers)

97. Answer A

   Diabetes

98. Answer C

   Loss of bladder or bowel control

99. Answer A

   A common disorder that affects the autonomic nervous system

100. Answer B

   Medications to manage symptoms.

MEDICAL ASSISTANT CERTIFICATION
EXAMINATION STUDY GUIDE
PART-NINE

1. What is high blood pressure?

    a. A medical condition where the force of blood against artery walls is low enough to cause

       health problems

    b. A medical condition where the force of blood against artery walls is high enough to cause

       health problems

    c. A medical condition where the force of blood against artery walls is normal.

    d. A medical condition where the force of blood against artery walls is irrelevant.

2. How long does it typically take for high blood pressure to develop?

    a. A few weeks

    b. A few months

    c. A few years

    d. It develops suddenly.

3. What are the health problems associated with uncontrolled high blood pressure?

    a. Headaches

    b. Dizziness

    c. Heart disease

    d. All of the above

4. Are signs or symptoms usually present in most people with high blood pressure?

    a. Yes

    b. No

5. What are the symptoms of early-stage high blood pressure?

    a. Headaches

    b. Dizziness

    c. Nosebleeds

    d. All of the above

6. At what stage do symptoms of high blood pressure usually occur?

    a. Early stage

    b. Severe or life-threatening stage

    c. Both A and B

    d. None of the above

7. What is primary (essential) hypertension?

    a. Hypertension is caused by an underlying condition.

    b. Hypertension with no identifiable cause

    c. Hypertension that develops suddenly

    d. None of the above

8. What is secondary hypertension?

    a. Hypertension is caused by an underlying condition.

    b. Hypertension with no identifiable cause

    c. Hypertension that develops suddenly

    d. None of the above

9. Which type of high blood pressure usually develops slowly over the course of many years?

    a. Primary (essential) hypertension

    b. Secondary hypertension

    c. Both A and B

    d. None of the above

10. Which type of high blood pressure usually appears suddenly and causes a higher blood pressure than primary hypertension?

    a. Primary (essential) hypertension

    b. Secondary hypertension

    c. Both A and B

    d. None of the above

11. What is the normal range for blood pressure?

    a. 80/60 mmHg

    b. 120/80 mmHg

    c. 140/90 mmHg

    d. 160/100 mmHg

12. What lifestyle changes can help control high blood pressure?

    a. Eating a healthy diet

    b. Regular exercise

    c. Quitting smoking

    d. All of the above

13. What is the recommended limit for daily sodium intake for people with high blood pressure?

    a. 1,500 mg

    b. 2,000 mg

    c. 2,500 mg

    d. 3,000 mg

14. What is the recommended limit for daily alcohol intake for men with high blood pressure?

    a. 1 drink per day

    b. 2 drinks per day

    c. 3 drinks per day

    d. 4 drinks per day

15. What is the recommended limit for daily alcohol intake for women with high blood pressure?

    a. 1 drink per day

    b. 2 drinks per day

    c. 3 drinks per day

    d. 4 drinks per day

16. What is the name of the device used to measure blood pressure?

    a. Thermometer

    b. Stethoscope

    c. Sphygmomanometer

    d. Otoscope

17. What is the top number in a blood pressure reading called?

    a. Diastolic pressure

    b. Systolic pressure

    c. Pulse pressure

    d. Mean arterial pressure.

18. What is the bottom number in a blood pressure reading called?

    a. Diastolic pressure

    b. Systolic pressure

    c. Pulse pressure

    d. Mean arterial pressure.

19. What is the term used to describe blood pressure that is consistently higher than normal but not yet in the high blood pressure range?

    a. Prehypertension

    b. Hypotension

    c. Hypertension crisis

    d. Malignant hypertension

20. What is the term used to describe a sudden and severe increase in blood pressure that can cause organ damage?

    a. Prehypertension

    b. Hypotension

    c. Hypertension crisis

    d. Malignant hypertension

21. What is the medical term for high blood pressure?

    a. Hypotension

    b. Hypertension

    c. Hypoxia

    d. Hyperglycemia

22. What is the most common type of high blood pressure?

    a. Primary hypertension

    b. Secondary hypertension

    c. Malignant hypertension

    d. Isolated systolic hypertension

23. What is the term used to describe high blood pressure that is caused by an underlying medical condition?

    a. Primary hypertension

    b. Secondary hypertension

    c. Malignant hypertension

    d. Isolated systolic hypertension

24. What is the term used to describe high blood pressure that is accompanied by organ damage?

    a. Primary hypertension

    b. Secondary hypertension

    c. Malignant hypertension

    d. Isolated systolic hypertension

25. What is the term used to describe high blood pressure that only affects the systolic reading?

    a. Primary hypertension

    b. Secondary hypertension

    c. Malignant hypertension

    d. Isolated systolic hypertension

26. What is the term used to describe a blood pressure reading that is higher than normal but not yet in the high blood pressure range?

    a. Hypertension

    b. Prehypertension

    c. Hypotension

    d. Malignant hypertension

27. What is the term used to describe a blood pressure reading that is consistently higher than normal and requires medical attention?

    a. Hypertension

    b. Prehypertension

    c. Hypotension

    d. Malignant hypertension

28. What is the term used to describe a blood pressure reading that is consistently lower than normal?

    a.   Hypertension

    b.   Prehypertension

    c.   Hypotension

    d.   Malignant hypertension

29. What is the term used to describe a sudden drop in blood pressure that can cause dizziness or fainting?

    a.   Hypertension

    b.   Prehypertension

    c.   Hypotension

    d.   Malignant hypertension

30. What is the term used to describe a blood pressure reading that is higher than normal due to stress or anxiety?

    a.   White coat hypertension

    b.   Masked hypertension

    c.   Resistant hypertension

    d.   Orthostatic hypertension

31. What is the recommended blood pressure range for adults according to the American Heart Association?

    a. Less than 120/80 mmHg

    b. Less than 130/80 mmHg

    c. Less than 140/90 mmHg

    d. Less than 150/100 mmHg

32. What lifestyle changes can help lower high blood pressure?

    a. Eating a healthy diet, exercising regularly, and quitting smoking

    b. Drinking more alcohol, eating more salt, and avoiding exercise

    c. Eating a high-fat diet, avoiding fruits and vegetables, and not getting enough sleep

    d. None of the above

33. What type of medication is commonly used to treat high blood pressure?

    a. Antibiotics

    b. Antidepressants

    c. Antihistamines

    d. Antihypertensives

34. What is the term used to describe high blood pressure that is difficult to control with medication?

    a. Resistant hypertension

    b. Malignant hypertension

    c. Secondary hypertension

    d. Isolated systolic hypertension

35. What is the term used to describe high blood pressure that occurs during pregnancy?

    a. Prehypertension

    b. Gestational hypertension

    c. Malignant hypertension

    d. Secondary hypertension

36. What is the term used to describe a sudden, severe increase in blood pressure that can cause a medical emergency?

    a. Hypertensive crisis

    b. Hypertensive urgency

    c. Hypertensive emergency

    d. Hypertensive shock

37. What is the term used to describe a blood pressure reading that is higher than normal when taken outside of a medical setting?

    a.   White coat hypertension

    b.   Masked hypertension

    c.   Resistant hypertension

    d.   Orthostatic hypertension

38. What is the term used to describe a blood pressure reading that drops when a person stands up?

    a.   White coat hypertension

    b.   Masked hypertension

    c.   Resistant hypertension

    d.   Orthostatic hypertension

39. What is the term used to describe a blood pressure reading that is consistently high at night but normal during the day?

    a.   Nocturnal hypertension

    b.   Diurnal hypertension

    c.   Resistant hypertension

    d.   Masked hypertension

40. What is the term used to describe a blood pressure reading that is consistently high despite taking multiple medications?

   a.   Resistant hypertension

   b.   Malignant hypertension

   c.   Secondary hypertension

   d.   Isolated systolic hypertension

41. Which of the following is a risk factor for high blood pressure?

   a.   Being underweight

   b.   Being physically active

   c.   Having a family history of low blood pressure

   d.   Being overweight or obese

42. Which gender tends to develop hypertension after menopause?

   a.   Men

   b.   Women

   c.   Both men and women equally

   d.   None of the above

43. Which race is more likely to develop high blood pressure at an earlier age?

    a. Whites

    b. Blacks

    c. Asians

    d. Hispanics

44. Which of the following is a risk factor for high blood pressure that tends to run in families?

    a. Age

    b. Race

    c. Physical inactivity

    d. Family history

45. Which of the following is a risk factor for high blood pressure that is associated with a higher heart rate?

    a. Age

    b. Race

    c. Physical inactivity

    d. Family history

46. Which of the following is a risk factor for high blood pressure that is associated with an increased need for oxygen supply and nutrients to the tissue?

    a. Age

    b. Race

    c. Physical inactivity

    d. Overweight or obesity

47. Which of the following is a risk factor for high blood pressure that is more common in men through early middle age?

    a. Age

    b. Race

    c. Family history

    d. Physical inactivity

48. Which of the following is a risk factor for high blood pressure that is associated with complications such as stroke and heart attack?

    a. Age

    b. Race

    c. Family history

    d. Physical inactivity

49. Which of the following is a risk factor for high blood pressure that is associated with a lack of physical activity?

    a. Age

    b. Race

    c. Family history

    d. Physical inactivity

50. Which of the following is a risk factor for high blood pressure that is associated with a stronger force on the arteries?

    a. Age

    b. Race

    c. Family history

    d. Physical inactivity

51. Which of the following is a risk factor for high blood pressure that can be improved through lifestyle changes?

    a. Age

    b. Race

    c. Family history

    d. Physical inactivity

52. Which of the following is a risk factor for high blood pressure that can be improved through a healthy diet?

   a. Age

   b. Race

   c. Family history

   d. Overweight or obesity

53. Which of the following is a risk factor for high blood pressure that can be improved through stress management techniques?

   a. Age

   b. Race

   c. Family history

   d. Physical inactivity

54. Which of the following is a risk factor for high blood pressure that can be improved through quitting smoking?

   a. Age

   b. Race

   c. Family history

   d. Physical inactivity

55. Which of the following is a risk factor for high blood pressure that can be improved through limiting alcohol consumption?

    a. Age

    b. Race

    c. Family history

    d. Overweight or obesity

56. Which of the following is a risk factor for high blood pressure that can be improved through medication?

    a. Age

    b. Race

    c. Family history

    d. Chronic kidney disease

57. Which of the following is a risk factor for high blood pressure that can be improved through reducing salt intake?

    a. Age

    b. Race

    c. Family history

    d. Physical inactivity

58. Which of the following is a risk factor for high blood pressure that can be improved through reducing caffeine intake?

   a. Age

   b. Race

   c. Family history

   d. Overweight or obesity

59. Which of the following is a risk factor for high blood pressure that can be improved through getting enough sleep?

   a. Age

   b. Race

   c. Family history

   d. Physical inactivity

60. Which of the following is a risk factor for high blood pressure that can be improved through managing diabetes?

   a. Age

   b. Race

   c. Family history

   d. Chronic kidney disease

61. Which of the following can immediately raise blood pressure temporarily?

    a. Eating too much salt

    b. Drinking too much alcohol

    c. Not getting enough sleep

    d. Being physically inactive

62. How can tobacco use contribute to high blood pressure?

    a. It can damage the lining on artery walls.

    b. It can cause arteries to widen, decreasing blood pressure.

    c. It can increase the amount of potassium in cells.

    d. It can decrease the amount of sodium in cells.

63. How does too much sodium in a diet contribute to high blood pressure?

    a. It causes the body to release hormones that raise blood flow and heart rate.

    b. It damages the lining on artery walls.

    c. It causes arteries to narrow, increasing blood pressure.

    d. It causes the body to retain fluid, increasing blood pressure.

64. How does too little potassium in a diet contribute to high blood pressure?

    a. It causes the body to release hormones that raise blood flow and heart rate.

    b. It damages the lining on artery walls.

    c. It causes arteries to narrow, increasing blood pressure.

    d. It allows too much sodium to accumulate in blood.

65. How can high levels of stress contribute to high blood pressure?

    a. It can cause arteries to widen, decreasing blood pressure.

    b. It can damage the lining on artery walls.

    c. It can cause the body to retain fluid, increasing blood pressure.

    d. It can lead to a temporary yet dramatic increase in blood pressure.

66. Which chronic condition can increase the risk of high blood pressure?

    a. High cholesterol

    b. Low cholesterol

    c. Low blood sugar

    d. High blood sugar

67. How can pregnancy contribute to high blood pressure?

    a. It can cause arteries to widen, decreasing blood pressure.

    b. It can damage the lining on artery walls.

    c. It can cause the body to retain fluid, increasing blood pressure.

    d. It can lead to a temporary yet dramatic increase in blood pressure.

68. How does alcohol consumption contribute to high blood pressure?

    a. It causes the body to release hormones that raise blood flow and heart rate.

    b. It damages the lining on artery walls.

    c. It causes arteries to narrow, increasing blood pressure.

    d. It can damage the heart over time.

69. How can secondhand smoke contribute to high blood pressure?

    a. It can cause arteries to widen, decreasing blood pressure.

    b. It can damage the lining on artery walls.

    c. It can cause the body to retain fluid, increasing blood pressure.

    d. It can lead to a temporary yet dramatic increase in blood pressure.

70. How can physical inactivity contribute to high blood pressure?

    a. It can cause arteries to widen, decreasing blood pressure.

    b. It can damage the lining on artery walls.

    c. It can cause the body to retain fluid, increasing blood pressure.

    d. It can lead to a temporary yet dramatic increase in blood pressure.

71. What are the goals for the treatment of high blood pressure?

    a. To eliminate all sodium and water from the body

    b. To reduce blood volume and open blood vessels

    c. To lower blood pressure to a healthy range

    d. To increase the workload on the heart

72. What is the first step in controlling high blood pressure?

    a. Taking medications

    b. Changing personal lifestyle

    c. Increasing sodium intake

    d. Decreasing physical activity

73. When are medications used to lower blood pressure?

    a.   Only when lifestyle changes are not efficient enough.

    b.   Only when blood pressure is extremely high.

    c.   Only when there are no other medical problems.

    d.   Only when the person is experiencing symptoms.

74. What do thiazide diuretics do?

    a.   Reduce the workload on the heart.

    b.   Open blood vessels

    c.   Help the body eliminate sodium and water.

    d.   Block the formation of a natural chemical that narrows blood vessels.

75. Are diuretics the only choice in high blood pressure medication?

    a.   Yes

    b.   No, but they are often the first choice.

    c.   No, but they are only used in extreme cases.

    d.   No, but they are only used in combination with beta blockers.

76. What do beta blockers do?

    a. Help the body eliminate sodium and water.

    b. Open blood vessels

    c. Reduce the workload on the heart and open blood vessels.

    d. Block the formation of a natural chemical that narrows blood vessels.

77. Do beta blockers work as well in blacks or in the elderly when prescribed alone?

    a. Yes

    b. No

    c. It depends on the stage of high blood pressure.

    d. It depends on the other medical problems present.

78. When are beta blockers effective?

    a. When prescribed alone

    b. When combined with a thiazide diuretic

    c. When combined with an ACE inhibitor

    d. When combined with an angiotensin II receptor blocker

79. What do ACE inhibitors do?

   a. Help the body eliminate sodium and water.

   b. Open blood vessels

   c. Block the formation of a natural chemical that narrows blood vessels.

   d. Block the action of a natural chemical that narrows blood vessels.

80. What do angiotensin II receptor blockers do?

   a. Help the body eliminate sodium and water.

   b. Open blood vessels

   c. Block the formation of a natural chemical that narrows blood vessels.

   d. Block the action of a natural chemical that narrows blood vessels.

81. Which medication is often the first choice in high blood pressure medication?

   a. Beta blockers

   b. ACE inhibitors

   c. Angiotensin II receptor blockers

   d. Thiazide diuretics

82. Which medication is effective when combined with a thiazide diuretic?

   a.   Beta blockers

   b.   ACE inhibitors

   c.   Angiotensin II receptor blockers

   d.   All of the above

83. Which medication is less effective in blacks or in the elderly when prescribed alone?

   a.   Beta blockers

   b.   ACE inhibitors

   c.   Angiotensin II receptor blockers

   d.   Thiazide diuretics

84. Which medication helps relax blood vessels by blocking the formation of a natural chemical that

   narrows blood vessels?

   a.   Beta blockers

   b.   ACE inhibitors

   c.   Angiotensin II receptor blockers

   d.   Thiazide diuretics

85. Which medication helps relax blood vessels by blocking the action, not the formation, of a natural chemical that narrows blood vessels?

   a. Beta blockers

   b. ACE inhibitors

   c. Angiotensin II receptor blockers

   d. Thiazide diuretics

86. Which medication is often prescribed for people with heart failure?

   a. Beta blockers

   b. ACE inhibitors

   c. Angiotensin II receptor blockers

   d. Thiazide diuretics

87. Which medication is often prescribed for people with diabetes?

   a. Beta blockers

   b. ACE inhibitors

   c. Angiotensin II receptor blockers

   d. Thiazide diuretics

88. Which medication is often prescribed for people with kidney disease?

    a. Beta blockers

    b. ACE inhibitors

    c. Angiotensin II receptor blockers

    d. Thiazide diuretics

89. Which medication is often prescribed for people with asthma?

    a. Beta blockers

    b. ACE inhibitors

    c. Angiotensin II receptor blockers

    d. Thiazide diuretics

90. Which medication can cause potassium levels to increase in the blood?

    a. Beta blockers

    b. ACE inhibitors

    c. Angiotensin II receptor blockers

    d. Thiazide diuretics

91. Which medication can cause potassium levels to decrease in the blood?

    a.   Beta blockers

    b.   ACE inhibitors

    c.   Angiotensin II receptor blockers

    d.   Thiazide diuretics

92. Which medication can cause dizziness or lightheadedness?

    a.   Beta blockers

    b.   ACE inhibitors

    c.   Angiotensin II receptor blockers

    d.   Thiazide diuretics

93. Which medication can cause a dry cough?

    a.   Beta blockers

    b.   ACE inhibitors

    c.   Angiotensin II receptor blockers

    d.   Thiazide diuretic

94. Which medication can cause swelling in the legs, ankles, or feet?

    a. Beta blockers

    b. ACE inhibitors

    c. Angiotensin II receptor blockers

    d. Thiazide diuretics

95. Which medication can cause a slow heart rate?

    a. Beta blockers

    b. ACE inhibitors

    c. Angiotensin II receptor blockers

    d. Thiazide diuretics

96. Which medication can cause impotence or sexual dysfunction?

    a. Beta blockers

    b. ACE inhibitors

    c. Angiotensin II receptor blockers

    d. Thiazide diuretics

97. Which medication can cause a rash or hives?

    a.   Beta blockers

    b.   ACE inhibitors

    c.   Angiotensin II receptor blockers

    d.   Thiazide diuretics

98. Which medication can cause fatigue or weakness?

    a.   Beta blockers

    b.   ACE inhibitors

    c.   Angiotensin II receptor blockers

    d.   Thiazide diuretics

99. Which medication can cause nausea or vomiting?

    a.   Beta blockers

    b.   ACE inhibitors

    c.   Angiotensin II receptor blockers

    d.   Thiazide diuretics

100. Which medication can cause a metallic taste in the mouth?

a. Beta blockers

b. ACE inhibitors

c. Angiotensin II receptor blockers

d. Thiazide diuretics

PART-NINE

ANSWER TO MEDICAL ASSISTANT QUESTIONS

1. Answer B.

    A medical condition where the force of blood against artery walls is high enough to cause health

    problems.

2. Answer C

    It typically takes many years for high blood pressure to develop.

3. Answer C

    Uncontrolled high blood pressure can lead to health problems such as heart disease.

4. Answer B

    Signs or symptoms are usually not present in most people with high blood pressure.

5. Answer D

    Headaches, dizziness, and nosebleeds can be symptoms of early-stage high blood pressure.

6. Answer B

    Symptoms of high blood pressure usually occur at a severe or life-threatening stage.

7. Answer B

    Primary (essential) hypertension is high blood pressure with no identifiable cause.

8. Answer A

    Secondary hypertension is high blood pressure caused by an underlying condition

9. Answer A

Primary (essential) hypertension usually develops slowly over many years.

10. Answer B

Secondary hypertension usually appears suddenly and causes a higher blood pressure than primary

hypertension.

11. Answer B

The normal range for blood pressure is 120/80 mmHg.

12. Answer D

Eating a healthy diet, regular exercise, and quitting smoking are all lifestyle changes that can help

control high blood pressure.

13. Answer A

The recommended limit for daily sodium intake for people with high blood pressure is 1,500 mg.

14. Answer A

The recommended limit for daily alcohol intake for men with high blood pressure is 1 drink per day.

15. Answer A

The recommended limit for daily alcohol intake for women with high blood pressure is 1 drink per

day.

16. Answer C

A sphygmomanometer is a device used to measure blood pressure.

17. Answer B

The top number in a blood pressure reading is called systolic pressure.

18. Answer A

The bottom number in a blood pressure reading is called diastolic pressure.

19. Answer A

Prehypertension is the term used to describe blood pressure that is consistently higher than normal

but not yet in the high blood pressure range.

20. Answer C

Hypertension crisis is the term used to describe a sudden and severe increase in blood pressure that

can cause organ damage.

21. Answer B

Hypertension is the medical term for high blood pressure.

22. Answer A

Primary hypertension is the most common type of high blood pressure, accounting for about 90-

95% of cases.

23. Answer B

Secondary hypertension is the term used to describe high blood pressure that is caused by an

underlying medical condition, such as kidney disease or sleep apnea.

24. Answer C

Malignant hypertension is the term used to describe high blood pressure that is accompanied by

organ damage, such as damage to the kidneys, eyes, or brain.

25. Answer D

Isolated systolic hypertension is the term used to describe high blood pressure that only affects the

systolic reading (the top number in a blood pressure reading).

26. Answer B

Prehypertension is the term used to describe a blood pressure reading that is higher than normal but

not yet in the high blood pressure range.

27. Answer A

Hypertension is the term used to describe a blood pressure reading that is consistently higher than

normal and requires medical attention.

28. Answer C

Hypotension is the term used to describe a blood pressure reading that is consistently lower than

normal.

29. Answer C

Hypotension is the term used to describe a sudden drop in blood pressure that can cause dizziness

or fainting.

30. Answer A

White coat hypertension is the term used to describe a blood pressure reading that is higher than

normal due to stress or anxiety, often in a medical setting (such as a doctor's office) where the patient

may feel nervous or anxious.

31. Answer B

Less than 130/80 mmHg is the recommended blood pressure range for adults according to the

American Heart Association.

32. Answer A

Eating a healthy diet, exercising regularly, and quitting smoking are lifestyle changes that can help

lower high blood pressure.

33. Answer D

Antihypertensives are medications commonly used to treat high blood pressure.

34. Answer A

Resistant hypertension is the term used to describe high blood pressure that is difficult to control

with medication.

35. Answer B

Gestational hypertension is the term used to describe high blood pressure that occurs during

Pregnancy

36. Answer C

Hypertensive emergency is the term used to describe a sudden, severe increase in blood pressure that can cause a medical emergency.

37. Answer B

Masked hypertension is the term used to describe a blood pressure reading that is higher than normal when taken outside of a medical setting.

38. Answer D

Orthostatic hypertension is the term used to describe a blood pressure reading that drops when a person stands up.

39. Answer A

Nocturnal hypertension is the term used to describe a blood pressure reading that is consistently high at night but normal during the day.

40. Answer A

Resistant hypertension is the term used to describe a blood pressure reading that is consistently high despite taking multiple medications.

41. Answer D

Being overweight or obese is a risk factor for high blood pressure because the more a person weighs, the more blood is needed for oxygen supply and nutrients to the tissue, which increases the pressure on the artery walls.

42. Answer B

Women tend to develop hypertension after menopause due to hormonal changes.

43. Answer B

Blacks are more likely to develop high blood pressure at an earlier age compared to whites.

44. Answer D

Family history is a risk factor for high blood pressure because it tends to run in families.

45. Answer C

Physical inactivity is a risk factor for high blood pressure because it can lead to a higher heart rate,

which increases the force on the arteries.

46. Answer D

Overweight or obesity is a risk factor for high blood pressure because it increases the need for

oxygen supply and nutrients to the tissue, which increases the pressure on the artery walls.

47. Answer A

Age is a risk factor for high blood pressure because the risk increases with age.

48. Answer B

Race is a risk factor for high blood pressure because it is more common among blacks and

complications such as stroke and heart attack are more common in blacks.

49. Answer D

   Physical inactivity is a risk factor for high blood pressure because it can lead to a higher heart rate

   and increase the risk of being overweight or obese.

50. Answer D

   Being overweight or obese is a risk factor for high blood pressure because it increases the pressure

   on the artery walls

51. Answer D

   Physical inactivity: Lack of physical activity or exercise is a risk factor for high blood pressure.

   Regular physical activity can help lower blood pressure.

52. Answer D

   Overweight or obesity: Being overweight or obese is a risk factor for high blood pressure. Losing

   weight through a healthy diet can help lower blood pressure.

53. Answer D

   Physical inactivity: Stress can cause temporary increases in blood pressure. Managing stress through

   techniques such as exercise, meditation, or deep breathing can help lower blood pressure.

54. Answer D

   Physical inactivity: Smoking can cause temporary increases in blood pressure. Quitting smoking can

   help lower blood pressure.

55. Answer A

Age: Drinking too much alcohol can raise blood pressure. Limiting alcohol consumption can help lower blood pressure.

56. Answer D

Chronic kidney disease: Some people with chronic kidney disease may need medication to help control their blood pressure.

57. Answer A

Age: Consuming too much salt can raise blood pressure. Reducing salt intake can help lower blood pressure.

58. Answer A

Age: Consuming too much caffeine can raise blood pressure. Reducing caffeine intake can help lower blood pressure.

59. Answer A

Age: Getting enough sleep is important for overall health, including blood pressure. Lack of sleep or poor quality sleep can raise blood pressure.

60. Answer D

Chronic kidney disease: People with diabetes are at higher risk for developing high blood pressure. Managing diabetes through medication and lifestyle changes can help lower blood pressure.

61. Answer B

Drinking too much alcohol: Drinking too much alcohol can immediately raise blood pressure temporarily, as it can cause the body to release hormones that raise blood flow and heart rate.

62. Answer A

It can damage the lining on artery walls: Tobacco use can immediately raise blood pressure temporarily and damage the lining on artery walls, which can cause arteries to narrow and increase blood pressure.

63. Answer D

It causes the body to retain fluid, increasing blood pressure: Too much sodium in a diet can cause the body to retain fluid, which increases blood pressure.

64. Answer D

It allows too much sodium to accumulate in blood: Too little potassium in a diet can allow too much sodium to accumulate in blood, which can increase blood pressure.

65. Answer D

It can lead to a temporary yet dramatic increase in blood pressure: High levels of stress can lead to a temporary yet dramatic increase in blood pressure.

66. Answer A

High cholesterol: Certain chronic conditions, such as high cholesterol, can increase the risk of high blood pressure.

67. Answer C

It can cause the body to retain fluid, increasing blood pressure: Pregnancy can contribute to high

blood pressure by causing the body to retain fluid, which increases blood pressure.

68. Answer D

It can damage the heart over time: Drinking too much alcohol can damage the heart over time,

which can contribute to high blood pressure.

69. Answer B

It can damage the lining on artery walls: Secondhand smoke can contribute to high blood pressure

by damaging the lining on artery walls.

70. Answer D

It can lead to a temporary yet dramatic increase in blood pressure: Physical inactivity can lead to a

temporary yet dramatic increase in blood pressure. Regular physical activity can help lower blood

pressure.

71. Answer C

To lower blood pressure to a healthy range: The goals for the treatment of high blood pressure are

to lower blood pressure to a healthy range.

72. Answer B

Changing personal lifestyle: The first step in controlling high blood pressure is changing personal

lifestyle.

73. Answer A

Only when lifestyle changes are not efficient enough: Medications are used to lower blood pressure

only when lifestyle changes are not efficient enough.

74. Answer C

Help the body eliminate sodium and water: Thiazide diuretics help the body eliminate sodium and

water and reduce blood volume.

75. Answer B

No, but they are often the first choice: Diuretics are not the only choice in high blood pressure

medication, but they are often the first choice.

76. Answer C

Reduce the workload on the heart and open blood vessels: Beta blockers reduce the workload on the

heart and open blood vessels, which cause the heart to beat slower and with less force.

77. Answer B

No: Beta blockers do not work as well in blacks or in the elderly when prescribed alone.

78. Answer B

When combined with a thiazide diuretic: Beta blockers are effective when combined with a thiazide

diuretic.

79. Answer C

Block the formation of a natural chemical that narrows blood vessels: ACE inhibitors help relax blood vessels by blocking the formation of a natural chemical that narrows blood vessels.

80. Answer D

   Block the action of a natural chemical that narrows blood vessels: Angiotensin II receptor blockers

   help relax blood vessels by blocking the action, not the formation, of a natural chemical that narrows

   blood vessels.

81. Answer D

   Thiazide diuretics: Thiazide diuretics are often the first choice in high blood pressure medication.

82. Answer D

   All of the above: Beta blockers, ACE inhibitors, and angiotensin II receptor blockers are effective

   when combined with a thiazide diuretic.

83. Answer A

   Beta blockers: Beta blockers are less effective in blacks or in the elderly when prescribed alone.

84. Answer B

   Block the formation of a natural chemical that narrows blood vessels: ACE inhibitors help relax

   blood vessels by blocking the formation of a natural chemical that narrows blood vessels.

85. Answer C

   Block the action of a natural chemical that narrows blood vessels: Angiotensin II receptor blockers.

   help relax blood vessels by blocking the action, not the formation, of a natural chemical that narrows

   blood vessels.

86. Answer B

ACE inhibitors: ACE inhibitors are often prescribed for people with heart failure because they help

relax blood vessels and reduce the workload on the heart.

87. Answer C

Angiotensin II receptor blockers: Angiotensin II receptor blockers are often prescribed for people

with diabetes because they help protect the kidneys and reduce the risk of kidney disease.

88. Answer B

ACE inhibitors: ACE inhibitors are often prescribed for people with kidney disease because they

help protect the kidneys and reduce the risk of further damage.

89. Answer D

Thiazide diuretics: Thiazide diuretics are often prescribed for people with asthma because they do

not cause bronchoconstriction, which can worsen asthma symptoms

90. Answer B

ACE inhibitors: ACE inhibitors can cause potassium levels to increase in the blood, which can be

dangerous if levels get too high.

91. Answer D

Thiazide diuretics: Thiazide diuretics can cause potassium levels to decrease in the blood, which can

be dangerous if levels get too low.

92. Answer A

Beta blockers: Beta blockers can cause dizziness or lightheadedness, especially when standing up quickly.

93. Answer B

ACE inhibitors: ACE inhibitors can cause a dry cough, which can be bothersome for some people.

94. Answer D

Thiazide diuretics: Thiazide diuretics can cause swelling in the legs, ankles, or feet, especially if taken in high doses.

95. Answer A

Beta blockers: Beta blockers can cause a slow heart rate, which can be dangerous for people with certain heart conditions.

96. Answer A

Beta blockers: Beta blockers can cause impotence or sexual dysfunction, which can be a concern for some people.

97. Answer C

Angiotensin II receptor blockers: Angiotensin II receptor blockers can cause a rash or hives, which can be a sign of an allergic reaction.

98. Answer D

Thiazide diuretics: Thiazide diuretics can cause fatigue or weakness, especially if taken in high doses.

99. Answer D

Thiazide diuretics: Thiazide diuretics can cause nausea or vomiting, especially if taken in high doses.

100.Answer D

Thiazide diuretics: Thiazide diuretics can cause a metallic taste in the mouth, which can be

bothersome for some people.

MEDICAL ASSISTANT CERTIFICATION
EXAMINATION STUDY GUIDE
PART-TEN

1. What is considered a normal blood pressure reading?

   a. 100/60 mmHg

   b. 120/80 mmHg

   c. 140/90 mmHg

   d. 160/100 mmHg

2. What is prehypertension?

   a. Systolic pressure of 120-139 mmHg or diastolic pressure of 80-89 mmHg

   b. Systolic pressure of 140-159 mmHg or diastolic pressure of 90-99 mmHg

   c. Systolic pressure of 160 mmHg or higher or diastolic pressure of 100 mmHg or higher

   d. None of the above

3. Which type of hypertension tends to get worse over time?

   a. Normal blood pressure

   b. Prehypertension

   c. Stage 1 hypertension

   d. Stage 2 hypertension

4. What is stage 1 hypertension?

   a. Systolic pressure of 120-139 mmHg or diastolic pressure of 80-89 mmHg

   b. Systolic pressure of 140-159 mmHg or diastolic pressure of 90-99 mmHg

   c. Systolic pressure of 160 mmHg or higher or diastolic pressure of 100 mmHg or higher

   d. None of the above

5. What is stage 2 hypertension?

    a. Systolic pressure of 120-139 mmHg or diastolic pressure of 80-89 mmHg

    b. Systolic pressure of 140-159 mmHg or diastolic pressure of 90-99 mmHg

    c. Systolic pressure of 160 mmHg or higher or diastolic pressure of 100 mmHg or higher

    d. None of the above

6. After the age of 50, which blood pressure reading is even more important?

    a. Systolic pressure

    b. Diastolic pressure

    c. Both systolic and diastolic pressure are equally important

    d. None of the above

7. What is a sphygmomanometer?

    a. A medical device used to measure blood pressure.

    b. A device used to measure heart rate.

    c. A device used to measure oxygen saturation in the blood.

    d. None of the above

8. What is the purpose of the inflatable cuff in a sphygmomanometer?

    a. To restrict blood flow

    b. To measure blood pressure

    c. To determine at what pressure blood flow is starting.

    d. None of the above

9. What is the purpose of the mercury manometer in a sphygmomanometer?

   a. To restrict blood flow

   b. To measure blood pressure

   c. To determine at what pressure blood flow is starting.

   d. None of the above

10. How is a manual sphygmomanometer used?

   a. In combination with a stethoscope

   b. In combination with an ECG machine

   c. In combination with an ultrasound machine

   d. None of the above

11. What are the components of a sphygmomanometer?

   a. Inflatable cuff, measuring unit, inflation bulb, and valve.

   b. Measuring unit, stethoscope, and valve

   c. Inflatable cuff, ECG machine, and valve

   d. None of the above

12. What is the purpose of the inflation bulb in a sphygmomanometer?

   a. To restrict blood flow

   b. To measure blood pressure

   c. To inflate the cuff

   d. None of the above

13. What is the purpose of the valve in a sphygmomanometer?

    a. To restrict blood flow

    b. To measure blood pressure

    c. To determine at what pressure blood flow is starting.

    d. To release air from the cuff

14. What is an aneroid gauge in a sphygmomanometer?

    a. A type of inflatable cuff

    b. A type of measuring unit

    c. A type of inflation bulb

    d. None of the above

15. Which blood pressure reading is considered prehypertension?

    a. Systolic pressure of 120-139 mmHg or diastolic pressure of 80-89 mmHg

    b. Systolic pressure of 140-159 mmHg or diastolic pressure of 90-99 mmHg

    c. Systolic pressure of 160 mmHg or higher or diastolic pressure of 100 mmHg or higher

    d. None of the above

16. What is the difference between systolic and diastolic blood pressure?

    a. Systolic pressure is the pressure in the arteries when the heart beats, while diastolic pressure is the pressure in the arteries when the heart is at rest.

    b. Systolic pressure is the pressure in the arteries when the heart is at rest, while diastolic pressure is the pressure in the arteries when the heart beats.

    c. Systolic pressure is the pressure in the veins when the heart beats, while diastolic pressure is the pressure in the veins when the heart is at rest.

    d. None of the above

17. What is the most common cause of hypertension?

    a. Genetics

    b. Poor diet

    c. Lack of exercise

    d. Stress

18. What are some lifestyle changes that can help manage hypertension?

    a. Eating a healthy diet, exercising regularly, quitting smoking, and reducing stress

    b. Taking medication, reducing caffeine intake, and getting enough sleep

    c. Drinking alcohol in moderation, reducing salt intake, and avoiding processed foods

    d. None of the above

19. What is the DASH diet?

    a. A diet that emphasizes fruits, vegetables, whole grains, lean proteins, and low-fat dairy products

    b. A diet that emphasizes high-fat foods and restricts carbohydrates.

    c. A diet that emphasizes high-protein foods and restricts carbohydrates.

    d. None of the above

20. What is the recommended daily sodium intake for individuals with hypertension?

    a. Less than 2,300 mg

    b. Less than 1,500 mg

    c. Less than 3,000 mg

    d. None of the above

21. What is the respiration rate considered to be tachypnea?

    a. Less than 12 breaths per minute

    b. Between 12 and 20 breaths per minute

    c. More than 20 breaths per minute

    d. None of the above

22. What are some causes of tachypnea?

    a. Heart or lung problems

    b. Panic attacks or anxiety

    c. Allergies or asthma

    d. All of the above

23. What is the difference between obstructive sleep apnea and central sleep apnea?

    a. Obstructive sleep apnea occurs when the airway is blocked, while central sleep apnea occurs when the brain fails to send the proper signals to the muscles that control breathing.

    b. Obstructive sleep apnea occurs when the brain fails to send the proper signals to the muscles that control breathing, while central sleep apnea occurs when the airway is blocked.

    c. Both obstructive sleep apnea and central sleep apnea occur when the airway is blocked.

    d. Both obstructive sleep apnea and central sleep apnea occur when the brain fails to send the proper signals to the muscles that control breathing.

24. What are some causes of apnea?

    a. Heart or lung problems

    b. Illegal drugs or certain medications

    c. Both A and B

    d. None of the above

25. What is the period of time called when breathing completely stops or is significantly reduced?

    a. Tachypnea

    b. Bradypnea

    c. Apnea

    d. None of the veu8

26. What is the respiration rate considered to be normal for an adult?

    a. Less than 12 breaths per minute

    b. Between 12 and 20 breaths per minute

    c. More than 20 breaths per minute

    d. None of the above

27. What is the term used to describe abnormally fast respiration rates?

    a. Tachypnea

    b. Bradypnea

    c. Apnea

    d. None of the above

28. What is the term used to describe abnormally slow respiration rates?

    a. Tachypnea

    b. Bradypnea

    c. Apnea

    d. None of the above

29. What are some causes of tachypnea?

    a. Heart or lung problems

    b. Panic attacks or anxiety

    c. Allergies or asthma

    d. All of the above

30. What are some causes of bradypnea?

    a. Heart or lung problems

    b. Illegal drugs or certain medications

    c. Both A and B

    d. None of the above

31. What is the respiration rate considered to be normal for an average healthy adult?

    a. Less than 10 breaths per minute

    b. Between 10 and 16 breaths per minute

    c. Between 16 and 20 breaths per minute

    d. More than 20 breaths per minute

32. When measuring the respiration rate, what position should the patient be in?

    a. Standing

    b. Sitting

    c. Lying down

    d. Any position is fine.

33. What is the range of normal respiration rate for smaller children (newborn to 6 years)?

    a. Less than 10 breaths per minute

    b. Between 10 and 16 breaths per minute

    c. Between 16 and 20 breaths per minute

    d. More than 20 breaths per minute

34. What is the heart rate also known as?

    a. Blood pressure

    b. Oxygen saturation

    c. Respiratory rate

    d. Pulse

35. How is the heart rate usually recorded?

    a. As mmHg

    b. As mL/min

    c. As bpm

    d. As L/min

36. When can a person's heart rate change?

    a. During eating

    b. During sleeping

    c. During watching TV

    d. None of the above

37. Where can a person's pulse be felt?

   a. Only at the wrist

   b. Only at the neck

   c. At any place that allows an artery to be compressed against a bone

   d. None of the above

38. How can the pulse be measured using a stethoscope?

   a. By listening to the heartbeat

   b. By measuring the blood pressure

   c. By measuring the oxygen saturation

   d. None of the above

39. What can the pulse be used to determine?

   a. A person's overall level of health

   b. A person's blood pressure

   c. A person's respiratory rate

   d. None of the above

40. What is considered to be a lower pulse rate?

   a. Less than 60 bpm

   b. Between 60 and 80 bpm

   c. Between 80 and 100 bpm

   d. More than 100 bpm

41. What is the condition called when the heart rate drops below 60 bpm?

    a. Tachycardia

    b. Bradycardia

    c. Arrhythmia

    d. None of the above

42. What is the term used to describe the pulse felt at the wrist?

    a. Carotid pulse

    b. Brachial pulse

    c. Radial pulse

    d. Popliteal pulse

43. What is the term used to describe the pulse felt at the neck?

    a. Carotid pulse

    b. Brachial pulse

    c. Radial pulse

    d. Popliteal pulse

44. What is the term used to describe the pulse felt behind the knee?

    a. Carotid pulse

    b. Brachial pulse

    c. Radial pulse

    d. Popliteal pulse

45. What is the term used to describe the pulse felt around the ankle joint?

    a. Carotid pulse

    b. Brachial pulse

    c. Radial pulse

    d. Posterior tibial pulse

46. What is the term used to describe difficulty breathing?

    a. Hypoxia

    b. Hypertension

    c. Hypotension

    d. Dyspnea

47. What is the term used to describe a rapid breathing rate?

    a. Bradypnea

    b. Tachypnea

    c. Apnea

    d. Hypopnea

48. What is the term used to describe a slow breathing rate?

    a. Bradypnea

    b. Tachypnea

    c. Apnea

    d. Hypopnea

49. What is the term used to describe the amount of air inhaled and exhaled with each breath?

    a. Tidal volume

    b. Vital capacity

    c. Residual volume

    d. Inspiratory reserve volume

50. What is the term used to describe the maximum amount of air that can be exhaled after a maximum inhalation?

    a. Tidal volume

    b. Vital capacity

    c. Residual volume

    d. Expiratory reserve volume

51. What is the term used to describe the amount of air that remains in the lungs after a maximum exhalation?

    a. Tidal volume

    b. Vital capacity

    c. Residual volume

    d. Inspiratory reserve volume

52. What is the term used to describe the amount of air that can be inhaled after a normal inhalation?

    a. Tidal volume

    b. Vital capacity

    c. Residual volume

    d. Inspiratory reserve volume

53. What is the term used to describe the amount of air that can be exhaled after a normal exhalation?

    a. Tidal volume

    b. Vital capacity

    c. Residual volume

    d. Expiratory reserve volume

54. What is the term used to describe the amount of air that can be inhaled after a forced exhalation?

    a. Tidal volume

    b. Vital capacity

    c. Residual volume

    d. Inspiratory reserve volume

55. What is the term used to describe the amount of air that can be exhaled after a forced inhalation?

    a. Tidal volume

    b. Vital capacity

    c. Residual volume

    d. Expiratory reserve volume

56. What is the natural occurrence during respiration where heart rate changes slightly while breathing in and then returns to normal?

    a. Emotional stress

    b. Physical stress

    c. Medication

    d. Breathing

57. What increases the heart rate as the heart has to beat faster and harder for more oxygen?

   a. Emotional stress

   b. Physical stress

   c. Medication

   d. Breathing

58. What causes hormones to be released that make the heart work harder to provide muscles with sufficient energy?

   a. Emotional stress

   b. Physical stress

   c. Medication

   d. Breathing

59. What can cause changes in the heart rate, including an increase in heart rate?

   a. Emotional stress

   b. Physical stress

   c. Medication

   d. Breathing

60. What can also slow down the heart rate?

   a. Emotional stress

   b. Physical stress

   c. Medication

   d. Breathing

61. What involves special sensors that will adjust to blood pressure changes?

    a. Vagal stimulation

    b. Emotional stress

    c. Physical stress

    d. Medication

62. What can cause an increase in heart rate?

    a. Digitalis preparations

    b. Beta blockers

    c. Stimulants

    d. Breathing

63. What can cause the heart rate to slow down?

    a. Emotional stress

    b. Physical stress

    c. Medication

    d. Vagal stimulation

64. What can cause an increase in heart rate if heart problems are not present?

    a. Emotional stress

    b. Physical stress

    c. Medication

    d. Breathing

65. What can cause the heart rate to slow down if heart problems are present?

    a. Emotional stress

    b. Physical stress

    c. Medication

    d. Breathing's

66. What may cause slight changes in heart rate, although a person may not notice this change as it may not be significant enough?

    a. Emotional stress

    b. Physical stress

    c. Medication

    d. Breathing

67. What can cause the heart rate to slow down due to increased oxygen need?

    a. Emotional stress

    b. Physical stress

    c. Medication

    d. Breathing

68. What can cause the heart to work harder to provide muscles with sufficient energy?

    a. Emotional stress

    b. Physical stress

    c. Medication

    d. Breathing

69. What can cause changes in the heart rate, including a slowing down of the heart rate?

    a. Emotional stress

    b. Physical stress

    c. Medication

    d. Vagal stimulation

70. What can cause an increase in heart rate due to the release of hormones?

    a. Emotional stress

    b. Physical stress

    c. Medication

    d. Breathing

71. What is vagal stimulation?

    a. A type of medication

    b. A type of heart surgery

    c. A process that adjusts to blood pressure changes

    d. A type of heart rhythm disorder

72. What happens to the heart rate during physical activities like lifting heavy objects or going through labor?

    a. It slows down.

    b. It speeds up.

    c. It remains the same.

    d. It becomes irregular.

73. What happens to the heart rate during illnesses like fever?

    a. It slows down.

    b. It speeds up.

    c. It remains the same.

    d. It becomes irregular.

74. What happens to the heart rate when the body can no longer fight an infection?

    a. It slows down.

    b. It speeds up.

    c. It remains the same.

    d. It becomes irregular.

75. What heart problems can be caused by plaque buildup in arteries?

    a. Heart attack

    b. Heart failure

    c. Arrhythmias

    d. All of the above

76. What are arrhythmias?

    a. Heart attacks

    b. Heart failures

    c. Irregular heart rhythms

    d. Plaque buildup in arteries

77. How does tachycardia affect the heart's efficiency?

    a. It pumps more efficiently.

    b. It pumps less efficiently.

    c. It remains the same.

    d. It becomes irregular.

78. What is the resting heart rate for bradycardia?

    a. More than 100 bpm

    b. 60 bpm or less

    c. 70-80 bpm

    d. 90-100 bpm

79. What can cause bradycardia?

    a. Not enough oxygen pumped to the heart.

    b. Plaque buildup in arteries

    c. Emotional stress

    d. Physical stress near

80. What are the symptoms of bradycardia?

    a. Shortness of breath

    b. Fainting

    c. Cardiac arrest

    d. All of the above

81. What is the definition of tachycardia?

    a. Resting heart rate of 60 bpm or less

    b. Resting heart rate of more than 100 bpm

    c. Irregular heart rhythms

    d. Plaque buildup in arteries

82. What is the definition of bradycardia?

    a. Resting heart rate of 60 bpm or less

    b. Resting heart rate of more than 100 bpm

    c. Irregular heart rhythms

    d. Plaque buildup in arteries

83. What can cause an increase in heart rate due to the release of hormones?

    a. Emotional stress

    b. Physical stress

    c. Medication

    d. Breathing

84. What can cause changes in the heart rate, including a slowing down of the heart rate?

    a. Emotional stress

    b. Physical stress

    c. Medication

    d. Breathing

85. What can cause the heart rate to slow down due to increased oxygen need?

    a. Emotional stress

    b. Physical stress

    c. Medication

    d. Breathing

86. What can cause an increase in heart rate if heart problems are not present?

    a. Emotional stress

    b. Physical stress

    c. Medication

    d. Breathing

87. What can cause the heart rate to slow down if heart problems are present?

    a. Emotional stress

    b. Physical stress

    c. Medication

    d. Breathing

88. What may cause slight changes in heart rate, although a person may not notice this change as it may not be significant enough?

    a. Emotional stress

    b. Physical stress

    c. Medication

    d. Breathing

89. What can cause the heart to work harder to provide muscles with sufficient energy?

    a. Emotional stress

    b. Physical stress

    c. Medication

    d. Breathing

90. What can also slow down the heart rate?

    a. Emotional stress

    b. Physical stress

    c. Medication

    d. Breathing techniques

91. What is the normal range for blood pressure in adults?

    a. 90/60 mmHg to 120/80 mmHg

    b. 120/80 mmHg to 140/90 mmHg

    c. 140/90 mmHg to 160/100 mmHg

    d. 160/100 mmHg to 180/110 mmHg

92. What is the medical term for high blood pressure?

    a. Hypertension

    b. Hypotension

    c. Hyperglycemia

    d. Hypoglycemia

93. What is the medical term for low blood pressure?

    a. Hypotension

    b. Hypertension

    c. Hyperglycemia

    d. Hypoglycemia

94. What is the normal range for heart rate in adults?

    a. 60 bpm to 100 bpm

    b. 50 bpm to 80 bpm

    c. 70 bpm to 120 bpm

    d. 80 bpm to 140 bpm

95. What is the medical term for a fast heart rate?

    a. Tachycardia

    b. Bradycardia

    c. Arrhythmia

    d. Atherosclerosis

96. What is the medical term for a slow heart rate?

    a. Bradycardia

    b. Tachycardia

    c. Arrhythmia

    d. Atherosclerosis

97. What is the medical term for an irregular heart rhythm?

    a. Arrhythmia

    b. Tachycardia

    c. Bradycardia

    d. Atherosclerosis

98. What is the medical term for a heart attack?

    a. Myocardial infarction

    b. Atherosclerosis

    c. Arrhythmia

    d. Hypertension

99. What is the medical term for a stroke?

    a. Cerebrovascular accident

    b. Myocardial infarction

    c. Atherosclerosis

    d. Arrhythmia

100. What is the medical term for a blood clot?

    a. Thrombus

    b. Embolus

    c. Aneurysm

    d. Hemorrhage

PART-TEN
ANSWER TO MEDICAL ASSISTANT QUESTIONS

1. Answer: B

   Blood pressure reading of 120/80 mmHg is considered normal.

2. Answer: A

   Prehypertension is a blood pressure reading where the systolic pressure ranges from 120 to 139 mmHg or diastolic pressure ranges from 80 to 89 mmHg.

3. Answer: B

   Prehypertension tends to get worse over time if not managed properly.

4. Answer: B

   Stage 1 hypertension is a blood pressure reading where the systolic pressure ranges from 140 to 159 mmHg or diastolic pressure ranges from 90 to 99 mmHg.

5. Answer: C

   Stage 2 hypertension is a blood pressure reading where the systolic pressure is 160 mmHg or higher or diastolic pressure is 100 mmHg or higher.

6. Answer: A

   After the age of 50, the systolic blood pressure reading is even more important than the diastolic blood pressure reading.

7. Answer: A

A sphygmomanometer is a medical device used to measure blood pressure.

8. Answer: A

The purpose of the inflatable cuff in a sphygmomanometer is to restrict blood flow.

9. Answer: B

The purpose of the mercury manometer in a sphygmomanometer is to measure blood pressure.

10. Answer: A

A manual sphygmomanometer is used in combination with a stethoscope.

11. Answer: A

The components of a sphygmomanometer include an inflatable cuff, a measuring unit.

12. Answer: C

The purpose of the inflation bulb in a sphygmomanometer is to inflate the cuff.

13. Answer: D

The purpose of the valve in a sphygmomanometer is to release air from the cuff.

14. Answer: B

An aneroid gauge is a type of measuring unit in a sphygmomanometer.

15. Answer: A

A blood pressure reading where the systolic pressure ranges from 120 to 139 mmHg or diastolic Pressure ranges from 80 to 89 mmHg is considered prehypertension.

16. Answer: A

Systolic pressure is the pressure in the arteries when the heart beats, while diastolic pressure is the

pressure in the arteries when the heart is at rest.

17. Answer: B

Poor diet is the most common cause of hypertension.

18. Answer: A

Eating a healthy diet, exercising regularly, quitting smoking, and reducing stress are some lifestyle

changes that can help manage hypertension.

19. Answer: A

The DASH diet is a diet that emphasizes fruits, vegetables, whole grains, lean proteins, and low-fat.

dairy products.

20. Answer: B

The recommended daily sodium intake for individuals with hypertension is less than 1,500 mg.

21. Answer: C

Respiration rate of more than 20 breaths per minute is considered tachypnea.

22. Answer: D

Tachypnea can be caused by heart or lung problems, panic attacks or anxiety, allergies, or asthma, or

other factors.

23. Answer: A

Obstructive sleep apnea occurs when the airway is blocked, while central sleep apnea occurs when the brain fails to send the proper signals to the muscles that control breathing.

24. Answer: C

Apnea can be caused by heart or lung problems, illegal drugs or certain medications, or other factors.

25. Answer: C

The period of time where breathing completely stops or is significantly reduced is called apnea.

26. Answer: B

The normal respiration rate for an adult is between 12 and 20 breaths per minute.

27. Answer: A

Tachypnea is the term used to describe abnormally fast respiration rates.

28. Answer: B

Bradypnea is the term used to describe abnormally slow respiration rates.

29. Answer: D

Tachypnea can be caused by heart or lung problems, panic attacks or anxiety, allergies, or asthma, or other factors.

30. Answer: C

Bradypnea can be caused by heart or lung problems, illegal drugs, or certain medications, or other. factors.

31. Answer: C

The respiration rate considered to be normal for an average healthy adult is between 16 and 20 breaths per minute.

32. Answer: C

The patient should be in a lying down position when measuring for respiration rate.

33. Answer: D

Smaller children (newborn to 6 years) breathe much faster, and a normal respiration rate for them is more than 20 breaths per minute.

34. Answer: D

The heart rate is also known as pulse.

35. Answer: C

The heart rate is usually recorded as bpm (beats per minute).

36. Answer: B

A person's heart rate can change during sleeping.

37. Answer: C

A person's pulse can be felt at any place that allows an artery to be compressed against a bone, such as the radial artery (wrist), the neck (carotid artery), the elbow inside (brachial artery), behind the knee (Popliteal artery) as well as around the ankle joint (posterior tibial artery).

38. Answer: A

The pulse can be measured using a stethoscope by listening directly to the heartbeat.

39. Answer: A

The pulse can be used to determine a person's overall level of health.

40. Answer: A

   In general, a lower pulse rate is considered better, and a pulse rate less than 60 bpm is considered lower.

41. Answer: B

   The condition called when the heart rate drops below 60 bpm is called bradycardia.

42. Answer: C

   The term used to describe the pulse felt at the wrist is radial pulse.

43. Answer: A

   The term used to describe the pulse felt at the neck is carotid pulse.

44. Answer: D

   The term used to describe the pulse felt behind the knee is popliteal pulse.

45. Answer: D

   The term used to describe the pulse felt around the ankle joint is posterior tibial pulse.

46. Answer: D

   Dyspnea is the medical term used to describe difficulty breathing or shortness of breath.

47. Answer B

   Tachypnea is the medical term used to describe a rapid breathing rate, typically greater than 20 breaths per minute in adults.

48. Answer: A

Bradypnea is the medical term used to describe a slow breathing rate, typically less than 12 breaths per minute in adults.

49. Answer: A

Tidal volume is the amount of air that is inhaled and exhaled with each breath during normal breathing.

50. Answer: B

Vital capacity is the maximum amount of air that can be exhaled after a maximum inhalation.

51. Answer: C

Residual volume is the amount of air that remains in the lungs after a maximum exhalation.

52. Answer: D

Inspiratory reserve volume is the amount of air that can be inhaled after a normal inhalation.

53. Answer: D

Expiratory reserve volume is the amount of air that can be exhaled after a normal exhalation.

54. Answer: D

Inspiratory reserve volume is the amount of air that can be inhaled after a forced exhalation.

55. Answer: B

Vital capacity is the maximum amount of air that can be exhaled after a maximum inhalation, including any additional air that can be exhaled after a forced inhalation.

56. Answer: D

Breathing is the natural occurrence during respiration where heart rate changes slightly while breathing

in and then returns to normal.

57. Answer: B.

Physical stress increases the heart rate as the heart has to beat faster and harder for more oxygen.

58. Answer: A.

Emotional stress causes hormones to be released that make the heart work harder to provide muscles

with sufficient energy.

59. Answer: C.

Medication can cause changes in the heart rate, including an increase in heart rate.

60. Answer: D.

Breathing can also slow down the heart rate.

61. Answer: A.

Vagal stimulation involves special sensors that will adjust to blood pressure changes.

62. Answer: C.

Stimulants can cause an increase in heart rate.

63. Answer: C

Medication can cause the heart rate to slow down.

64. Answer: B.

Physical stress can cause an increase in heart rate if heart problems are not present.

65. Answer: B

Physical stress can cause the heart rate to slow down if heart problems are present.

66. Answer: D.

Breathing may cause slight changes in heart rate, although a person may not notice this change as it may not be significant enough.

67. Answer: B.

Physical stress can cause the heart rate to slow down due to increased oxygen need.

68. Answer: A.

Emotional stress can cause the heart to work harder to provide muscles with sufficient energy

69. Answer: C.

Dedication can cause changes in the heart rate, including a slowing down of the heart rate.

70. Answer: A.

Emotional stress can cause an increase in the heart rate due to the release of hormones.

71. Answer C.

A process that adjusts to blood pressure changes

Vagal stimulation is a process that involves special sensors that adjust to blood pressure changes.

72. Answer A

It slows down.

During physical activities like lifting heavy objects or going through labor, the higher blood pressure

will signal the heart to slow down.

73. Answer B.

It speeds up during illnesses like fever, the heart rate increases due to increased oxygen requirements.

74. Answer A

It slows down. If the body can no longer fight an infection, the circulatory system crashes and heart

rate drops.

75. Answer D.

All of the above

Heart problems caused by plaque buildup in arteries (atherosclerosis) can lead to heart attack, failure

of the heart or irregular heart rhythms (arrhythmias).

76. Answer C.

Irregular heart rhythms

Arrhythmias are irregular heart rhythms that may affect the heart rate, either increasing it or decreasing

it.

77. Answer B.

It pumps less efficiently.

As the heart beats faster, it pumps less efficiently and less blood flow is provided to the body,

including the heart.

78. Answer B
   60 bpm or less
   Bradycardia is defined as a resting heart rate of 60 bpm or less.

79. Answer A
   Not enough oxygen pumped to the heart.
   Bradycardia can be caused when not enough oxygen is pumped to the heart and can therefore result in cardiac arrest.

80. Answer D.

   All of the above

   Bradycardia can result in shortness of breath, fainting or even death.

81. Answer A

   Resting heart rate of more than 100 bpm

   Tachycardia is defined as a resting heart rate of more than 100 bpm.

82. Answers A

   Resting heart rate of 60 bpm or less

   Bradycardia is defined as a resting heart rate of 60 bpm or less.

83. Answer A.

   Emotional stress

   Emotional stress can cause an increase in the heart rate due to the release of hormones.

84. Answer C

   Medication

   Medication can cause changes in the heart rate, including a slowing down of the heart rate.

85. Answer B

    Physical stress

    Physical stress can cause the heart rate to slow down due to increased oxygen need.

86. Answer B.

    Physical stress

    Physical stress can cause an increase in heart rate if heart problems are not present.

87. Answer B

    Physical stress

    Physical stress can cause the heart rate to slow down if heart problems are present.

88. Answer D.

    Breathing

    Breathing may cause slight changes in heart rate, although a person may not notice this change as it
    may not be significant enough.

89. Answer B

    Physical stress

    Physical stress can cause the heart to work harder to provide muscles with sufficient energy.

90. Answer C

    Medication

    Medication can also slow down the heart rate.

91. Answer A.

   60 mmHg to 120/80 mmHg

   The normal range for blood pressure in adults is between 90/60 mmHg to 120/80 mmHg.

92. Answer A.

   Hypertension

   The medical term for high blood pressure is hypertension.

93. Answer A

   Hypotension

   The medical term for low blood pressure is hypotension.

94. Answers A

   A. 60 bpm to 100 bpm

   The normal range for heart rate in adults is between 60 bpm to 100 bpm.

95. Answer A

   Tachycardia

   The medical term for a fast heart rate is tachycardia.

96. Answer A

   Bradycardia

   The medical term for a slow heart rate is bradycardia.

97. Answer A

   The medical term for an irregular heart rhythm is arrhythmia.

98. Answers A

   Myocardial infarction

   The medical term for a heart attack is myocardial infarction.

99. Answer A

   Cerebrovascular accident

   The medical term for a stroke is cerebrovascular accident.

100.Answer A

   Thrombus

   The medical term for a blood clot is thrombus.

MEDICAL ASSISTANT CERTIFICATION
EXAMINATION STUDY GUIDE
PART-ELEVEN

1. What is a person's heart rate defined by?

    a. Blood pressure

    b. Respiratory rate

    c. Pulse of the body

    d. Body temperature

2. Which fingers are used to feel the pulse?

    a. Thumb and index finger

    b. Index finger and middle finger

    c. Middle finger and ring finger

    d. Ring finger and pinky finger

3. Which artery is located in the wrist and commonly used to measure pulse?

    a. Ulnar artery

    b. Carotid artery

    c. Brachial artery

    d. Radial artery

4. What is an EKG used for?

    a. To measure blood pressure

    b. To measure respiratory rate

    c. To measure heart problems or heart disease

    d. To measure body temperature

5. What is the record produced by an EKG called?

    a. Electrocardiogram

    b. Electroencephalogram

    c. Electromyogram

    d. Electroneurogram

6. Which pulse site is located in the groin area?

    a. Ulnar pulse

    b. Radial pulse

    c. Femoral pulse

    d. Popliteal pulse

7. Which pulse site is located on the top of the foot?

    a. Popliteal pulse

    b. Tibialis posterior pulse

    c. Femoral pulse

    d. Dorsalis pedis pulse

8. Which pulse site is located on the side of the neck?

    a. Ulnar pulse

    b. Radial pulse

    c. Brachial pulse

    d. Carotid pulse

9. Which pulse site is located behind the knee?

    a. Ulnar pulse

    b. Radial pulse

    c. Popliteal pulse

    d. Dorsalis pedis pulse

10. Which pulse site is located on the inside of the elbow?

    a. Ulnar pulse

    b. Radial pulse

    c. Brachial pulse

    d. Carotid pulse

11. Which artery is located in the abdomen and is not commonly used to measure pulse?

    a. Ulnar artery

    b. Carotid artery

    c. Brachial artery

    d. Abdominal aorta

12. Which pulse site is located on the inside of the ankle?

    a.   Popliteal pulse

    b.   Tibialis posterior pulse

    c.   Femoral pulse

    d.   Dorsalis pedis pulse

13. What is the normal range for resting heart rate in adults?

    a.   30-50 beats per minute

    b.   60-100 beats per minute

    c.   120-150 beats per minute

    d.   180-200 beats per minute

14. What is the medical term for an abnormally slow heart rate?

    a.   Tachycardia

    b.   Bradycardia

    c.   Arrhythmia

    d.   Fibrillation

15. What is the medical term for an irregular heart rhythm?

    a.   Tachycardia

    b.   Bradycardia

    c.   Arrhythmia

    d.   Fibrillation

16. What is the medical term for a rapid heart rate?

    a.   Tachycardia

    b.   Bradycardia

    c.   Arrhythmia

    d.   Fibrillation

17. What is the medical term for a quivering or irregular heartbeat?

    a.   Tachycardia

    b.   Bradycardia

    c.   Arrhythmia

    d.   Fibrillation

18. What is the medical term for a heart rate that is faster than normal?

    a.   Tachycardia

    b.   Bradycardia

    c.   Arrhythmia

    d.   Fibrillation

19. What is the medical term for a heart rate that is slower than normal?

    a.   Tachycardia

    b.   Bradycardia

    c.   Arrhythmia

    d.   Fibrillation

20. What is the medical term for a heart rate that is irregular or abnormal?

    a. Tachycardia

    b. Bradycardia

    c. Arrhythmia

    d. Fibrillation

21. Which of the following is not a common method for measuring heart rate?

    a. Pulse oximetry

    b. Electrocardiogram (ECG)

    c. Blood pressure cuff

    d. Stethoscope

22. Which of the following is a non-invasive method for measuring heart rate?

    a. Cardiac catheterization

    b. Holter monitor

    c. Echocardiogram

    d. Pulse oximetry

23. Which of the following is a device used to measure heart rate during exercise?

    a. Holter monitor

    b. Echocardiogram

    c. Treadmill stress test

    d. Cardiac catheterization

24. Which of the following is a method for measuring heart rate that involves attaching electrodes to the chest?

    a.   Pulse oximetry

    b.   Electrocardiogram (ECG)

    c.   Blood pressure cuff

    d.   Stethoscope

25. Which of the following is a method for measuring heart rate that involves wearing a device that records heart activity over a period of time?

    a.   Pulse oximetry

    b.   Electrocardiogram (ECG)

    c.   Holter monitor

    d.   Stethoscope

26. What is the average weight of an adult brain?

    a.   1 pound

    b.   2 pounds

    c.   3 pounds

    d.   4 pounds

27. What is the function of the spinal cord?

    a.   To control actions of the body

    b.   To relay information from and to the brain

    c.   To separate the brain from the skull

    d.   To support the vertebral column

28. How long is the spinal cord?

    a. About 1 inch

    b. About 8 inches

    c. About 16 inches

    d. About 27 inches

29. How many segments does the spinal cord consist of?

    a. 8

    b. 12

    c. 16

    d. 31

30. Which part of the nervous system is the brain a part of?

    a. Central nervous system

    b. Peripheral nervous system

    c. Autonomic nervous system

    d. Enteric nervous system

31. What separates the brain from the skull?

    a. Neurons

    b. Glia

    c. Meninges

    d. Vertebral column

32. How does the brain develop over time?

    a. It grows in size

    b. It develops new neurons

    c. It develops new glia

    d. It develops through experience and learning

33. How many spinal nerves exit from each segment of the spinal cord?

    a. 1

    b. 2

    c. 3

    d. 4

34. Which part of the nervous system is responsible for controlling involuntary actions such as breathing and heart rate?

    a. Central nervous system

    b. Peripheral nervous system

    c. Autonomic nervous system

    d. Enteric nervous system

35. Which part of the nervous system is responsible for controlling voluntary movements such as walking and talking?

    a. Central nervous system

    b. Peripheral nervous system

    c. Autonomic nervous system

    d. Enteric nervous system

36. Which part of the nervous system is responsible for transmitting sensory information from the body to the brain?

    a. Central nervous system

    b. Peripheral nervous system

    c. Autonomic nervous system

    d. Enteric nervous system

37. Which part of the nervous system is responsible for transmitting motor information from the brain to the muscles?

    a. Central nervous system

    b. Peripheral nervous system

    c. Autonomic nervous system

    d. Enteric nervous system

38. Which part of the nervous system is responsible for controlling the digestive system?

    a. Central nervous system

    b. Peripheral nervous system

    c. Autonomic nervous system

    d. Enteric nervous system

39. Which part of the nervous system is responsible for controlling reflexes?

    a. Central nervous system

    b. Peripheral nervous system

    c. Autonomic nervous system

    d. Enteric nervous system

40. Which part of the nervous system is responsible for controlling the fight or flight response?

    a. Central nervous system

    b. Peripheral nervous system

    c. Autonomic nervous system

    d. Enteric nervous system

41. Which part of the nervous system is responsible for controlling the body's response to stress?

    a. Central nervous system

    b. Peripheral nervous system

    c. Autonomic nervous system

    d. Enteric nervous system

42. Which part of the nervous system is responsible for controlling the body's temperature?

    a. Central nervous system

    b. Peripheral nervous system

    c. Autonomic nervous system

    d. Enteric nervous system

43. Which part of the nervous system is responsible for controlling the body's sleep and wake cycles?

    a. Central nervous system

    b. Peripheral nervous system

    c. Autonomic nervous system

    d. Enteric nervous system

44. Which part of the nervous system is responsible for controlling the body's balance and coordination?

    a. Central nervous system

    b. Peripheral nervous system

    c. Autonomic nervous system

    d. Enteric nervous system

45. Which part of the nervous system is responsible for controlling the body's immune response?

    a. Central nervous system

    b. Peripheral nervous system

    c. Autonomic nervous system

    d. Enteric nervous system

46. Which part of the brain is responsible for regulating basic bodily functions such as breathing and heart rate?

    a. Cerebellum

    b. Medulla oblongata

    c. Thalamus

    d. Hypothalamus

47. Which part of the brain is responsible for processing visual information?

    a. Cerebellum

    b. Medulla oblongata

    c. Thalamus

    d. Occipital lobe

48. Which part of the brain is responsible for processing auditory information?

    a.   Cerebellum

    b.   Medulla oblongata

    c.   Thalamus

    d.   Temporal lobe

49. Which part of the brain is responsible for controlling voluntary movement?

    a.   Cerebellum

    b.   Medulla oblongata

    c.   Thalamus

    d.   Motor cortex

50. Which part of the brain is responsible for processing and interpreting sensory information?

    a.   Cerebellum

    b.   Medulla oblongata

    c.   Thalamus

    d.   Sensory cortex

51. Which part of the peripheral nervous system is responsible for voluntary control of body movements?

    a.   Autonomic nervous system

    b.   Sympathetic nervous system

    c.   Parasympathetic nervous system

    d.   Somatic nervous system

52. How many pairs of spinal nerves are there in the peripheral nervous system?

    a. 12

    b. 24

    c. 31

    d. 42

53. Which part of the autonomic nervous system is responsible for mobilizing the body's resources under stress?

    a. Sympathetic nervous system

    b. Parasympathetic nervous system

    c. Enteric nervous system

    d. Somatic nervous system

54. Which part of the autonomic nervous system is responsible for stimulating activities occurring while the body is under rest, including digestion and sexual arousal?

    a. Sympathetic nervous system

    b. Parasympathetic nervous system

    c. Enteric nervous system

    d. Somatic nervous system

55. Which part of the autonomic nervous system is responsible for controlling the gastrointestinal system?

    a. Sympathetic nervous system

    b. Parasympathetic nervous system

    c. Enteric nervous system

    d. Somatic nervous system

56. Which part of the peripheral nervous system sends sensory information to the central nervous system?

    a. Autonomic nervous system

    b. Sympathetic nervous system

    c. Parasympathetic nervous system

    d. Somatic nervous system

57. Which part of the peripheral nervous system projects motor nerve fibers to the skeletal muscle?

    a. Autonomic nervous system

    b. Sympathetic nervous system

    c. Parasympathetic nervous system

    d. Somatic nervous system

58. Which part of the autonomic nervous system controls smooth muscle of the internal organs and glands?

    a. Sympathetic nervous system

    b. Parasympathetic nervous system

    c. Enteric nervous system

    d. Somatic nervous system

59. Which part of the autonomic nervous system is responsible for lacrimation (tear production)?

    a. Sympathetic nervous system

    b. Parasympathetic nervous system

    c. Enteric nervous system

    d. Somatic nervous system

60. Which part of the autonomic nervous system is responsible for the fight or flight response?

    a. Sympathetic nervous system

    b. Parasympathetic nervous system

    c. Enteric nervous system

    d. Somatic nervous system

61. Which part of the autonomic nervous system is responsible for the rest and digest response?

    a. Sympathetic nervous system

    b. Parasympathetic nervous system

    c. Enteric nervous system

    d. Somatic nervous system

62. Which part of the peripheral nervous system carries information in the form of nerve impulses from the spinal cord to the body and back?

    a. Autonomic nervous system

    b. Sympathetic nervous system

    c. Parasympathetic nervous system

    d. Somatic nervous system

63. Which part of the autonomic nervous system is responsible for controlling the heart rate and blood pressure?

    a. Sympathetic nervous system

    b. Parasympathetic nervous system

    c. Enteric nervous system

    d. Somatic nervous system

64. Which part of the autonomic nervous system is responsible for controlling the constriction and dilation of the pupils?

   a. Sympathetic nervous system

   b. Parasympathetic nervous system

   c. Enteric nervous system

   d. Somatic nervous system

65. Which part of the autonomic nervous system is responsible for controlling the release of adrenaline and noradrenaline?

   a. Sympathetic nervous system

   b. Parasympathetic nervous system

   c. Enteric nervous system

   d. Somatic nervous system

66. Which part of the autonomic nervous system is responsible for controlling the secretion of saliva?

   a. Sympathetic nervous system

   b. Parasympathetic nervous system

   c. Enteric nervous system

   d. Somatic nervous system

67. Which part of the peripheral nervous system is responsible for carrying information from the body's sensory receptors to the central nervous system?

   a. Autonomic nervous system

   b. Sympathetic nervous system

   c. Parasympathetic nervous system

   d. Somatic nervous system

68. Which part of the autonomic nervous system is responsible for controlling the contraction and relaxation of the bladder?

    a.   Sympathetic nervous system

    b.   Parasympathetic nervous system

    c.   Enteric nervous system

    d.   Somatic nervous system

69. Which part of the autonomic nervous system is responsible for controlling the secretion of digestive enzymes and acid?

    a.   Sympathetic nervous system

    b.   Parasympathetic nervous system

    c.   Enteric nervous system

    d.   Somatic nervous system

70. Which part of the autonomic nervous system is responsible for controlling the constriction and dilation of the blood vessels?

    a.   Sympathetic nervous system

    b.   Parasympathetic nervous system

    c.   Enteric nervous system

    d.   Somatic nervous system

71. Which part of the eye is responsible for focusing light on the retina?

    a.   Cornea

    b.   Iris

    c.   Pupil

    d.   Optic nerve

72. Which part of the eye is responsible for detecting color?

    a. Rods

    b. Cones

    c. Optic nerve

    d. Cornea

73. Which part of the eye is responsible for detecting light?

    a. Rods

    b. Cones

    c. Optic nerve

    d. Cornea

74. Which part of the ear is responsible for transmitting vibrations to the inner ear?

    a. Outer ear

    b. Middle ear

    c. Inner ear

    d. Eardrum

75. Which part of the ear is responsible for reacting to vibrations and transmitting impulses to the brain?

    a. Outer ear

    b. Middle ear

    c. Inner ear

    d. Eardrum

76. Which part of the nose is responsible for detecting smells?

   a. Mucous membranes

   b. Sinuses

   c. Nasal cavity

   d. Olfactory bulb

77. What is the name of the chart used to determine a person's vision?

   a. Snellen Chart

   b. Eye Chart

   c. Vision Chart

   d. Sight Chart

78. What is the normal vision for the average person considered to be?

   a. 10/10

   b. 20/20

   c. 30/30

   d. 40/40

79. What is the term used to describe a constant buzzing or whistling sound in the ears?

   a. Tinnitus

   b. Vertigo

   c. Deafness

   d. Hearing loss

80. What is the term used to describe a refractive error caused by an abnormal shape of the lens or length of the eye?

    a. Farsightedness

    b. Nearsightedness

    c. Astigmatism

    d. Presbyopia

81. Which part of the eye is responsible for controlling the amount of light that enters the eye?

    a. Cornea

    b. Iris

    c. Pupil

    d. Optic nerve

82. Which part of the ear is responsible for amplifying sound waves?

    a. Outer ear

    b. Middle ear

    c. Inner ear

    d. Eardrum

83. Which part of the nose is responsible for transmitting signals to the brain about the smells detected by the mucous membranes?

    a. Sinuses

    b. Nasal cavity

    c. Olfactory bulb

    d. Mucous membranes

84. What is the term used to describe a refractive error where distant objects appear blurry?

    a.   Farsightedness

    b.   Nearsightedness

    c.   Astigmatism

    d.   Presbyopia

85. What is the term used to describe a refractive error where close objects appear blurry?

    a.   Farsightedness

    b.   Nearsightedness

    c.   Astigmatism

    d.   Presbyopia

86. What is cataract?

    a.   Clouding of the eye lens

    b.   Inflammation of the eye

    c.   Loss of vision in one eye

    d.   Eye infection

87. What are the symptoms of cataract?

    a.   Sensitivity to glare, double vision, color intensity loss or blurry vision

    b.   Redness, itching, and discharge from the eye

    c.   Pain and swelling in the eye

    d.   None of the above

88. How is cataract diagnosed?

    a.   Blood test

    b.   Urine test

    c.   Standard eye exam

    d.   X-ray

89. What is epilepsy?

    a.   A brain disorder that causes repeated seizures

    b.   A heart condition that causes chest pain

    c.   A lung condition that causes difficulty breathing

    d.   A skin condition that causes rashes

90. What causes epilepsy?

    a.   Brain injury, infections, dementia, brain tumor or metabolism disorders

    b.   Heart disease, high blood pressure, and high cholesterol

    c.   Lung disease, smoking, and air pollution

    d.   Skin infections and allergies

91. What is the most common type of seizure in epilepsy?

    a.   Focal (partial) seizures

    b.   Petit mal (absence) seizures

    c.   Grand mal (generalized tonic-clonic) seizures

    d.   All of the above

92. How is epilepsy diagnosed?

    a.   Blood test

    b.   Urine test

    c.   EEG (electroencephalogram)

    d.   X-ray

93. What is glaucoma?

    a.   A group of eye conditions causing damage to the optic nerve

    b.   A lung condition causing difficulty breathing

    c.   A heart condition causing chest pain

    d.   A skin condition causing rashes

94. What is the second most common cause of blindness in the US?

    a.   Cataract

    b.   Epilepsy

    c.   Glaucoma

    d.   None of the above

95. How many main types of glaucoma are there?

    a.   One

    b.   Two

    c.   Three

    d.   Four

96. Which type of glaucoma is the most common?

   a.   Chronic (open angle) glaucoma

   b.   Congenital glaucoma

   c.   Acute (angle closure) glaucoma

   d.   Secondary glaucoma

97. What are the symptoms of glaucoma?

   a.   Gradual loss of peripheral vision, tunnel vision, eye pain, and nausea

   b.   Sensitivity to glare, double vision, color intensity loss or blurry vision

   c.   Staring spells or dramatic seizures

   d.   None of the above

98. How is glaucoma diagnosed?

   a.   Blood test

   b.   Urine test

   c.   Standard eye exam

   d.   Tonometry test

99. What is the treatment for glaucoma?

   a.   Eyeglasses, magnifying glasses or changes in lighting

   b.   Medication and/or surgery

   c.   Antibiotics

   d.   None of the above

100. What is the best way to prevent cataracts, epilepsy, and glaucoma?

    a.   Eating a healthy diet and exercising regularly

    b.   Wearing protective eyewear and avoiding head injuries

    c.   Getting regular eye exams and seeking medical attention for seizures

    d.   All of the above

PART-ELEVEN

ANSWER TO MEDICAL ASSISTANT QUESTIONS

1. Answer: C

   Pulse of the body

2. Answer: B

   Index finger and middle finger

3. Answer: D

   Radial artery

4. Answer: C

   To measure heart problems or heart disease

5. Answer: A

   Electrocardiogram

6. Answer: C

   Femoral pulse

7. Answer: D

   Dorsalis pedis pulse

8. Answer: D

   Carotid pulse

9. Answer: C

   Popliteal pulse10. Answer: C

   Brachial pulse

11. Answer: D

   Abdominal aorta

12. Answer: B

   Tibialis posterior pulse

13. Answer: B

   60-100 beats per minute

14. Answer: B

   Bradycardia

15. Answer: C

   Arrhythmia

16. Answer: A

   Tachycardia

17. Answer: D

   Fibrillation

18. Answer: A

   Tachycardia

19. Answer: B

   Bradycardia

20. Answer: C

   Arrhythmia

21. Answer: C

   Blood pressure cuff

22. Answer D

   Pulse oximetry

23. Answer: C

   Treadmill stress test

24. Answer: B

   Electrocardiogram (ECG)

25. Answer: C

   Holter monitor

26. Answer: C

   3 pounds

27. Answer: B

   To relay information from and to the brain

28. Answer: C

   About 16 inches

29. Answer: D

   31

30. Answer: A

   Central nervous system

31. Answer: C

   Meninges

32. Answer: D

   It develops through experience and learning

33. Answer: A

   1

34. Answer: C

   Autonomic nervous system

35. Answer: A

    Central nervous system

36. Answer: B

    Peripheral nervous system

37. Answer: B

    Peripheral nervous system

38. Answer: D

    Enteric nervous system

39. Answer: A

    Central nervous system

40. Answer: C

    Autonomic nervous system

41. Answer: C

    Autonomic nervous system

42. Answer: C

    Autonomic nervous system

43. Answer: A

    Central nervous system

44. Answer: A
    Central nervous system

45. Answer: A

    Central nervous system

46. Answer: B

    Medulla oblongata

47. Answer: D

Occipital lobe

48. Answer: D

Temporal lobe

49. Answer: D

Motor cortex

50. Answer: D

Sensory cortex

51. Answer: D

Somatic nervous system

52. Answer: C

31

53. Answer: A

Sympathetic nervous system

54. Answer: B

Parasympathetic nervous system

55. Answer: C

Enteric nervous system

56. Answer: D

Somatic nervous system

57. Answer: D

Somatic nervous system

58. Answer: A

   Sympathetic nervous system

59. Answer: B

   Parasympathetic nervous system

60. Answer: A

   Sympathetic nervous system

61. Answer: B

   Parasympathetic nervous system

62. Answer:

   Somatic nervous system

63. Answer: A

   Sympathetic nervous system

64. Answer: A

   Sympathetic nervous system

65. Answer: A

   Sympathetic nervous system

66. Answer: B

   Parasympathetic nervous system

67. Answer: D

   Somatic nervous system

68. Answer: B

   Parasympathetic nervous system

69. Answer: B

   Parasympathetic nervous system

70. Answer: A

   Sympathetic nervous system

71. Answer: A

   Cornea

72. Answer: B

   Cones

73. Answer: A

   Rods

74. Answer: A

   Outer ear

75. Answer: C

   Inner ear

76. Answer: A

   Mucous membranes

77. Answer: A

   Snellen Chart

78. Answer: B

   20/20

79. Answer: A

   Tinnitus

80. Answer: C

   Astigmatism

81. Answer: B

   Iris

82. Answer: B

   Middle ear

83. Answer: C

   Olfactory bulb

84. Answer: B

   Nearsightedness

85. Answer: A

   Farsightedness

86. Answer: A

   Clouding of the eye lens

87. Answer: A

   Sensitivity to glare, double vision, color intensity loss or blurry vision

88. Answer: C

   Standard eye exam

89. Answer: A

   A brain disorder that causes repeated seizures

90. Answer: A

   Brain injury, infections, dementia, brain tumor or metabolism disorders

91. Answer: A

    Focal (partial) seizures

92. Answer: C

    EEG (electroencephalogram)

93. Answer: A

    A group of eye conditions causing damage to the optic nerve

94. Answer: C

    Glaucoma

95. Answer: D

    Four

96. Answer: A

    Chronic (open angle) glaucoma

97. Answer: A

    Gradual loss of peripheral vision, tunnel vision, eye pain, and nausea

98. Answer: D

    Tonometry test

99. Answer: B)

    Medication and/or surgery

100.Answer: D

    All of the above

MEDICAL ASSISTANT CERTIFICATION
EXAMINATION STUDY GUIDE
PART-TWELVE

1. What is the term for the act of breathing?

    a. Expiration

    b. Inhalation

    c. Respiration

    d. None of the above

2. Which of the following is not part of the upper respiratory tract?

    a. Nose

    b. Larynx

    c. Lungs

    d. Nasal cavity

3. Which of the following is not a sinus in the upper respiratory tract?

    a. Frontal sinus

    b. Maxillary sinus

    c. Sphenoidal sinus

    d. Bronchial sinus

4. Which of the following is not part of the lower respiratory tract?

    a. Lungs

    b. Bronchi

    c. Trachea

    d. Nasal cavity

5. Which organ is responsible for filtering, warming, and moistening the air we breathe?

   a. Nose

   b. Lungs

   c. Trachea

   d. Bronchi

6. Which organ is also known as the voice box?

   a. Nose

   b. Larynx

   c. Trachea

   d. Bronchi

7. Which organ is also known as the windpipe?

   a. Nose

   b. Larynx

   c. Trachea

   d. Bronchi

8. Which organ is responsible for the exchange of gases between the air and the blood?

   a. Nose

   b. Lungs

   c. Trachea

   d. Bronchi

9. Which part of the respiratory system is responsible for carrying air to the lungs?

   a. Nose

   b. Larynx

   c. Trachea

   d. Bronchi

10. Which part of the respiratory system is responsible for removing carbon dioxide from the body?

   a. Nose

   b. Lungs

   c. Trachea

   d. Bronchi

11. Air can enter the nose through which structure?

   a. Nasal conchae

   b. Vestibule

   c. Pharynx

   d. Larynx

12. What divides the nasal cavity into two parts?

   a. Nasal conchae

   b. Nasal septum

   c. Pharynx

   d. Larynx

13. Which bones form the walls of the nasal cavity?

   a. Nasal, frontal, and maxillary bones

   b. Nasal, frontal, maxillary, ethmoid, and sphenoid bones

   c. Nasal and maxillary bones

   d. Nasal and frontal bones

14. What forms the nasal floor?

   a. Nasal septum

   b. Palates

   c. Nasal conchae

   d. Vestibule

15. What is the external part of the nose made of?

   a. Cartilage

   b. Bone

   c. Muscle

   d. Ligament

16. What are the three areas of the pharynx?

   a. Upper, middle, and lower

   b. Nasal, oropharynx, and laryngopharynx

   c. Vestibule, nasopharynx, and oropharynx

   d. Larynx, trachea, and bronchi

17. What type of epithelium lines the pharynx?

    a. Simple squamous

    b. Stratified squamous

    c. Pseudostratified columnar

    d. Transitional

18. What is located in the posterior wall of the nasopharynx?

    a. Pharyngeal tonsils

    b. Palates

    c. Nasal conchae

    d. Vestibule

19. What is the function of the oropharynx?

    a. Passage for airflow coming from the nasal cavity

    b. Passage for food and air

    c. Passage for air only

    d. None of the above

20. What is the function of the larynx?

    a. To join the pharynx with the trachea

    b. To filter, warm, and moisten the air we breathe

    c. To exchange gases between the air and the blood

    d. None of the above

21. What is the function of the cartilages in the larynx?

    a.   To filter, warm, and moisten the air we breathe

    b.   To exchange gases between the air and the blood

    c.   To protect the vocal cords

    d.   None of the above

22. What is the name of the structure that connects the larynx to the trachea?

    a.   Nasal septum

    b.   Pharynx

    c.   Epiglottis

    d.   Cricoid cartilage

23. What is the function of the trachea?

    a.   To filter, warm, and moisten the air we breathe

    b.   To exchange gases between the air and the blood

    c.   To carry air to the lungs

    d.   None of the above

24. What is the name of the structure that divides the trachea into two bronchi?

    a.   Nasal septum

    b.   Pharynx

    c.   Epiglottis

    d.   Carina

25. What is the function of the bronchi?

    a. To filter, warm, and moisten the air we breathe

    b. To exchange gases between the air and the blood

    c. To carry air to the lungs

    d. None of the above

26. What is the name of the smallest branches of the bronchi?

    a. Bronchioles

    b. Alveoli

    c. Capillaries

    d. Trachea

27. What is the function of the alveoli?

    a. To filter, warm, and moisten the air we breathe

    b. To exchange gases between the air and the blood

    c. To carry air to the lungs

    d. None of the above

28. What is the name of the membrane that surrounds the lungs?

    a. Pleura

    b. Pericardium

    c. Peritoneum

    d. Epithelium

29. What is the function of the diaphragm?

    a. To filter, warm, and moisten the air we breathe

    b. To exchange gases between the air and the blood

    c. To carry air to the lungs

    d. To help with breathing by contracting and relaxing

30. What is the name of the muscle that helps with breathing?

    a. Diaphragm

    b. Trachea

    c. Bronchi

    d. Alveoli

31. What is the name of the process by which oxygen and carbon dioxide are exchanged between the lungs and the blood?

    a. Respiration

    b. Inhalation

    c. Exhalation

    d. Ventilation

32. What is the name of the condition in which the airways become inflamed and narrow, making it difficult to breathe?

    a. Asthma

    b. Bronchitis

    c. Pneumonia

    d. Emphysema

33. What is the name of the condition in which the air sacs in the lungs are damaged, making it difficult to breathe?

   a. Asthma

   b. Bronchitis

   c. Pneumonia

   d. Emphysema

34. What is the name of the condition in which the lungs become inflamed and filled with fluid, making it difficult to breathe?

   a. Asthma

   b. Bronchitis

   c. Pneumonia

   d. Emphysema

35. What is the name of the condition in which the bronchial tubes become inflamed and produce excess mucus, making it difficult to breathe?

   a. Asthma

   b. Bronchitis

   c. Pneumonia

   d. Emphysema

36. What is the name of the device used to measure lung function?

   a. Spirometer

   b. Stethoscope

   c. Otoscope

   d. Sphygmomanometer

37. What is the name of the process by which oxygen and carbon dioxide are transported in the blood?

    a. Diffusion

    b. Osmosis

    c. Active transport

    d. Passive transport

38. What is the name of the protein in red blood cells that carries oxygen?

    a. Hemoglobin

    b. Myoglobin

    c. Collagen

    d. Elastin

39. What is the name of the condition in which the body does not get enough oxygen?

    a. Hypoxia

    b. Hyperoxia

    c. Anoxia

    d. Asphyxia

40. What is the name of the condition in which the body has too much carbon dioxide?

    a. Hypercapnia

    b. Hypocapnia

    c. Anoxia

    d. Asphyxia

41. What is the function of the larynx?

    a. To filter, warm, and moisten the air we breathe

    b. To exchange gases between the air and the blood

    c. To protect the vocal cords

    d. None of the above

42. What is the name of the cartilage that closes the larynx during swallowing?

    a. Thyroid cartilage

    b. Epiglottis

    c. Cricoid cartilage

    d. Corniculate cartilage

43. What is the function of coughing?

    a. To exchange gases between the air and the blood

    b. To protect from irritants or foreign objects

    c. To carry air to the lungs

    d. None of the above

44. What is the lining of the trachea made of?

    a. Simple squamous epithelium

    b. Stratified squamous epithelium

    c. Pseudostratified ciliated columnar epithelium

    d. Transitional epithelium

45. What holds the tracheal cartilages together?

    a.   Tracheal muscle

    b.   Smooth muscle

    c.   Skeletal muscle

    d.   Cardiac muscle

46. What is the name of the smallest passages in the respiratory system?

    a.   Bronchi

    b.   Alveoli

    c.   Capillaries

    d.   Trachea

47. How many lobes does the right lung have?

    a.   One

    b.   Two

    c.   Three

    d.   Four

48. What is the name of the slit in the lung where lymphatics, nerves, and bronchial tubes reach the lung?

    a.   Apex

    b.   Hilus

    c.   Pleura

    d.   Bronchioles

49. What is the name of the condition in which the airways become inflamed and narrow, making it difficult to breathe?

    a. Asthma

    b. Bronchitis

    c. Pneumonia

    d. Emphysema

50. What is the name of the protein in red blood cells that carries oxygen?

    a. Hemoglobin

    b. Myoglobin

    c. Collagen

    d. Elastin

51. What is apnea?

    a. A condition where breathing has slowed or completely stopped

    b. A condition where the airways become inflamed and narrow

    c. A condition where the lungs are unable to expand properly

    d. A condition where the heart is unable to pump blood effectively

52. What are some common causes of apnea?

    a. Allergies and sinus infections

    b. High blood pressure and diabetes

    c. Asthma and pneumonia

    d. Choking and drug overdose

53. What is the treatment for asthma?

    a. Antibiotics

    b. Bronchodilators

    c. Antihistamines

    d. Painkillers

54. What is acute bronchitis?

    a. A condition caused by smoking and emphysema

    b. A condition caused by bacteria or virus

    c. A condition where the airways become inflamed and narrow

    d. A condition where breathing has slowed or completely stopped

55. What is chronic bronchitis?

    a. A condition caused by smoking and emphysema

    b. A condition caused by bacteria or virus

    c. A condition where the airways become inflamed and narrow

    d. A condition where breathing has slowed or completely stopped

56. What are the symptoms of bronchitis?

    a. Chest pain and shortness of breath

    b. Coughing and/or coughing up excessive mucus

    c. Wheezing and difficulty breathing

    d. All of the above

57. What is diphtheria?

    a.   A condition caused by smoking and emphysema

    b.   A condition caused by bacteria or virus

    c.   A condition where the airways become inflamed and narrow

    d.   A condition where breathing has slowed or completely stopped

58. How does diphtheria spread?

    a.   Through contaminated food and water

    b.   Through physical contact with an infected person

    c.   Through respiratory drops of coughing or sneezing

    d.   Through insect bites

59. What are the symptoms of diphtheria?

    a.   Coloration of the skin and heavy cough

    b.   Drooling and difficulties breathing

    c.   Rapid breathing and fever

    d.   All of the above

60. What is the treatment for apnea?

    a.   Antibiotics

    b.   Painkillers

    c.   Artificial respiration

    d.   Antihistamines

61. What is the most common cause of pneumonia?

    a.   Fungal infection

    b.   Bacterial infection

    c.   Viral infection

    d.   All of the above

62. What is the most common cause of sinusitis?

    a.   Bacterial infection

    b.   Fungal infection

    c.   Viral infection

    d.   None of the above

63. What is the most common symptom of scarlet fever?

    a.   Nasal congestion

    b.   Rash

    c.   Shortness of breath

    d.   None of the above

64. How is pneumonia diagnosed?

    a.   Blood test

    b.   Urine test

    c.   Physical examination and X-ray of the chest

    d.   None of the above

65. What is the age group with the highest incidence of tuberculosis?

    a. 0-5 years

    b. 6-14 years

    c. 15-30 years

    d. 31-50 years

66. What is the most common cause of scarlet fever?

    a. Fungal infection

    b. Bacterial infection

    c. Viral infection

    d. All of the above

67. What is the most common symptom of sinusitis?

    a. Rash

    b. Sore throat

    c. Shortness of breath

    d. None of the above

68. How is scarlet fever diagnosed?

    a. Blood test

    b. Urine test

    c. Physical examination or throat cultures

    d. None of the above

69. What is the treatment for tuberculosis?

    a. Antibiotics

    b. Allergy shots

    c. Nasal sprays

    d. None of the above

70. What is the difference between acute and chronic sinusitis?

    a. Acute sinusitis is caused by allergies, while chronic sinusitis is caused by bacterial infection

    b. Acute sinusitis lasts less than 4 weeks, while chronic sinusitis lasts more than 12 weeks

    c. Acute sinusitis is treated with nasal sprays, while chronic sinusitis is treated with antibiotics

    d. None of the above

71. What is the function of the circulatory system?

    a. To pass nutrients and hormones to and from the cells

    b. To maintain homeostasis and stabilize pH and body temperature

    c. To fight disease

    d. All of the above

72. What are the components of the circulatory system?

    a. Pulmonary circulation, systemic circulation, coronary circulation, closed cardiovascular system, and the heart

    b. Respiratory system, digestive system, and nervous system

    c. Muscular system, skeletal system, and integumentary system

    d. None of the above

73. What is the function of the pulmonary circulation?

    a. To carry oxygen-rich blood from the heart to the lungs

    b. To carry oxygen-depleted blood from the heart to the lungs

    c. To carry oxygen-rich blood from the lungs to the heart

    d. To carry oxygen-depleted blood from the lungs to the heart

74. Where does blood enter the right atrium in the pulmonary circulation?

    a. Pulmonary veins

    b. Pulmonary arteries

    c. Aorta

    d. None of the above

75. What is the function of the pulmonary veins in the pulmonary circulation?

    a. To carry oxygen-rich blood from the heart to the lungs

    b. To carry oxygen-depleted blood from the heart to the lungs

    c. To carry oxygen-rich blood from the lungs to the heart

    d. To carry oxygen-depleted blood from the lungs to the heart

76. What is the function of the systemic circulation?

    a. To carry oxygen-rich blood from the heart to the body

    b. To carry oxygen-depleted blood from the heart to the body

    c. To carry oxygen-rich blood from the body to the heart

    d. To carry oxygen-depleted blood from the body to the heart

77. Which circulation is longer, pulmonary or systemic?

    a.   Pulmonary

    b.   Systemic

    c.   They are the same length

    d.   None of the above

78. What is the function of the aorta in the systemic circulation?

    a.   To carry oxygen-rich blood from the heart to the body

    b.   To carry oxygen-depleted blood from the heart to the body

    c.   To carry oxygen-rich blood from the body to the heart

    d.   To carry oxygen-depleted blood from the body to the heart

79. What is the closed cardiovascular system?

    a.   The system of blood vessels that carry blood throughout the body

    b.   The system of blood vessels that carry blood to and from the lungs

    c.   The system of blood vessels that carry blood to and from the heart

    d.   None of the above

80. What is the function of the heart in the circulatory system?

    a.   To pump blood throughout the body

    b.   To carry oxygen-rich blood to the lungs

    c.   To carry oxygen-depleted blood from the lungs

    d.   None of the above

81. What is the tricuspid valve?

   a. A valve that separates the left atrium and left ventricle

   b. A valve that separates the right atrium and right ventricle

   c. A valve that separates the pulmonary artery and aorta

   d. None of the above

82. What is the mitral valve?

   a. A valve that separates the left atrium and left ventricle

   b. A valve that separates the right atrium and right ventricle

   c. A valve that separates the pulmonary artery and aorta

   d. None of the above

83. What is coronary circulation?

   a. The circulation of blood to and from the lungs

   b. The circulation of blood to and from the heart muscle

   c. The circulation of blood to and from the body

   d. None of the above

84. What is the function of the circulatory system in maintaining homeostasis?

   a. To regulate body temperature

   b. To regulate pH levels

   c. To regulate blood pressure

   d. All of the above

85. What is the function of blood cells in the circulatory system?

    a.   To carry oxygen and nutrients to the cells

    b.   To remove waste products from the cells

    c.   To fight infection and disease

    d.   All of the above

86. What is the function of the muscular system?

    a.   To provide balance to the body

    b.   To provide strength to the body

    c.   To provide posture to the body

    d.   All of the above

87. How many groups of muscles are there in the muscular system?

    a.   One

    b.   Two

    c.   Three

    d.   Four

88. What are the three groups of muscles in the muscular system?

    a.   Cardiac, smooth, and skeletal

    b.   Respiratory, digestive, and nervous

    c.   Muscular, skeletal, and integumentary

    d.   None of the above

89. How many muscles are there in the human body?

    a.   Over 100

    b.   Over 300

    c.   Over 600

    d.   Over 1000

90. What controls skeletal muscles?

    a.   ANS (autonomic nervous system)

    b.   CNS (central nervous system)

    c.   SNS (somatic nervous system)

    d.   None of the above

91. What is the shape of skeletal muscle fibers?

    a.   Cylindrical

    b.   Elongated and thin

    c.   Round

    d.   None of the above

92. What is the function of smooth muscles?

    a.   To produce movement

    b.   To form the muscle layers in the walls of internal organs

    c.   To control the heart

    d.   None of the above

93. How many nuclei do smooth muscles have?

    a. None

    b. One

    c. Two

    d. Three

94. What controls cardiac muscles?

    a. ANS (autonomic nervous system)

    b. CNS (central nervous system)

    c. SNS (somatic nervous system)

    d. None of the above

95. What is the shape of smooth muscles?

    a. Cylindrical

    b. Elongated and thin

    c. Round

    d. None of the above

96. What is the connective tissue that binds skeletal muscle fibers together?

    a. Tendons

    b. Ligaments

    c. Cartilage

    d. None of the above

97. What is the function of smooth muscles in the walls of arteries and veins?

   a. To regulate blood pressure

   b. To regulate blood sugar levels

   c. To regulate body temperature

   d. None of the above

98. What is the function of cardiac muscles?

   a. To produce movement

   b. To form the muscle layers in the walls of internal organs

   c. To control the heart

   d. None of the above

99. What is the function of the autonomic nervous system in controlling muscles?

   a. To control voluntary movements

   b. To control involuntary movements

   c. To control both voluntary and involuntary movements

   d. None of the above

100.What is the difference between skeletal and smooth muscles?

   a. Skeletal muscles are controlled by the ANS, while smooth muscles are controlled by the SNS

   b. Skeletal muscles are striated, while smooth muscles are not

   c. Skeletal muscles have only one nucleus, while smooth muscles have many

   d. None of the above

PART-TWELVE

ANSWER TO MEDICAL ASSISTANT QUESTIONS

1. Answer: C

    Respiration

2. Answer: C

    Lungs

3. Answer: D

    Bronchial sinus

4. Answer: D

    Nasal cavity

5. Answer: A

    Nose

6. Answer: B

    Larynx

7. Answer: C

    Trachea

8. Answer: B

    Lungs

9. Answer: D

    Bronchi

10. Answer: B

    Lungs

11. Answer: B

    Vestibule

12. Answer: B

    Nasal septum

13. Answer: B

    Nasal, frontal, maxillary, ethmoid, and sphenoid bones

14. Answer: B

    Palates

15. Answer: ACartilage

16. Answer: A

    Upper, middle, and lower

17. Answer: B

    Stratified squamous

18. Answer: A

    Pharyngeal tonsils

19. Answer: B

    Passage for food and air

20. Answer: A

    To join the pharynx with the trachea

21. Answer: C

    To protect the vocal cords

22. Answer: D

    Cricoid cartilage

23. Answer: C

    To carry air to the lungs

24. Answer: D

    Carina

25. Answer: C

    To carry air to the lungs

26. Answer: A

    Bronchioles

27. Answer: B

    To exchange gases between the air and the blood

28. Answer: A

    Pleura

29. Answer: D

    To help with breathing by contracting and relaxing

30. Answer: A

    Diaphragm

31. Answer: A

    Respiration

32. Answer: A

    Asthma

33. Answer: D

    Emphysema

34. Answer: C

    Pneumonia

35. Answer: B

    Bronchitis

36. Answer: A

    Spirometer

37. Answer: A

    Diffusion

38. Answer: A

    Hemoglobin

39. Answer: A

    Hypoxia

40. Answer: A

    Hypercapnia

41. Answer: C

    To protect the vocal cords

42. Answer: B

    Epiglottis

43. Answer: B

    To protect from irritants or foreign objects

44. Answer: C

    Pseudostratified ciliated columnar epithelium

45. Answer: A

    Tracheal muscle

46. Answer: B

    Alveoli

47. Answer: C

    Three

48. Answer: B

    Hilus

49. Answer: A

    Asthma

50. Answer: A

    Hemoglobin

51. Answer: A

    A condition where breathing has slowed or completely stopped

52. Answer: D

Choking and drug overdose

53. Answer: B

Bronchodilators

54. Answer: B

A condition caused by bacteria or virus

55. Answer: A

A condition caused by smoking and emphysema

56. Answer: B

Coughing and/or coughing up excessive mucus

57. Answer: B

A condition caused by bacteria or virus

58. Answer: C

Through respiratory drops of coughing or sneezing

59. Answer: D

All of the above

60. Answer: C

Artificial respiration

61. Answer: B

Bacterial infection

62. Answer: C

Viral infection

63. Answer: B

Rash

64. Answer: C

Physical examination and X-ray of the chest

65. Answer: C

15-30 years

66. Answer: B

Bacterial infection

67. Answer: B

    Sore throat

68. Answer: C

    Physical examination or throat cultures

69. Answer: A

    Antibiotics

70. Answer: B

    Acute sinusitis lasts less than 4 weeks, while chronic sinusitis lasts more than 12 weeks

71. Answer: D

    All of the above

72. Answer: A

    Pulmonary circulation, systemic circulation, coronary circulation, closed cardiovascular system, and the heart

73. Answer: B

    To carry oxygen-depleted blood from the heart to the lungs

74. Answer: B

    Pulmonary arteries

75. Answer: C

    To carry oxygen-rich blood from the lungs to the heart

76. Answer: A

    To carry oxygen-rich blood from the heart to the body

77. Answer: B

    Systemic

78. Answer: A

    To carry oxygen-rich blood from the heart to the body

79. Answer: A

    The system of blood vessels that carry blood throughout the body

80. Answer: A

    To pump blood throughout the body

81. Answer: B

    A valve that separates the right atrium and right ventricle

82. Answer: A

    A valve that separates the left atrium and left ventricle

83. Answer: B

    The circulation of blood to and from the heart muscle

84. Answer: D

    All of the above

85. Answer: D

    All of the above

86. Answer: D

    All of the above

87. Answer: C

    Three

88. Answer: A

    Cardiac, smooth, and skeletal

89. Answer: C

    Over 600

90. Answer: C

    SNS (somatic nervous system)

91. Answer: A

    Cylindrical

92. Answer: B

    To form the muscle layers in the walls of internal organs

93. Answer: B

    One

94. Answer: A

    ANS (autonomic nervous system)

95. Answer: B

    Elongated and thin

96. Answer: A

    Tendons

97. Answer: A

    To regulate blood pressure

98. Answer: C

    To control the heart

99. Answer: B

    To control involuntary movements

100. Answer: B

    Skeletal muscles are striated, while smooth muscles are not

MEDICAL ASSISTANT CERTIFICATION
EXAMINATION STUDY GUIDE
PART-THIRTEEN

1. What is the main component of bones that makes them hard and resistant to compression?

    a. Organic connective tissue

    b. Water

    c. Inorganic salts

    d. Blood vessels

2. What is the function of the skeletal system?

    a. To regulate body temperature

    b. To produce hormones

    c. To support other organs and anchor muscles

    d. To transport oxygen

3. Which type of bone protects the brain?

    a. Long bone

    b. Flat bone

    c. Irregular bone

    d. Pneumatic bone

4. What is the strength of bones comparable to?

    a. Rubber

    b. Glass

    c. Steel and iron

    d. Plastic

5. What type of bone is the patella (kneecap)?

    a. Long bone

    b. Flat bone

    c. Irregular bone

    d. Sesamoid bone

6. What is the function of tendons in the skeletal system?

    a. To support other organs

    b. To anchor muscles to bones

    c. To protect vital organs

    d. To regulate body temperature

7. What is the difference between compact bone and spongy bone?

    a. Compact bone is harder than spongy bone

    b. Spongy bone is denser than compact bone

    c. Compact bone is found in the ends of long bones, while spongy bone is found in the middle

    d.. Spongy bone contains more blood vessels than compact bone

8. What type of bone is the vertebrae?

    a. Long bone

    b. Flat bone

    c. Irregular bone

    d. Pneumatic bone

9. What is the function of ligaments in the skeletal system?

    a. To support other organs

    b. To anchor muscles to bones

    c. To protect vital organs

    d. To connect bones to other bones

10. What type of bone is the sternum (breastbone)?

    a. Long bone

    b. Flat bone

    c. Irregular bone

    d. Pneumatic bone

11. What is the main function of osteoblasts?

    a. To break down bone tissue

    b. To form new bone tissue

    c. To maintain bone matrix

    d. To regulate calcium levels in the blood

12. What is osteoid composed of?

   a. Type 1 collagen

   b. Type 2 collagen

   c. Type 3 collagen

   d. Type 4 collagen

13. What is the function of alkaline phosphatase in bone formation?

   a. To break down bone tissue

   b. To form new bone tissue

   c. To maintain bone matrix

   d. To regulate calcium levels in the blood

14. What is the main function of osteocytes?

   a. To break down bone tissue

   b. To form new bone tissue

   c. To maintain bone matrix

   d. To regulate calcium levels in the blood

15. What are the areas that osteocytes fill called?

   a. Canaliculi

   b. Lacunae

   c. Resorption pits

   d. Osteons

16. What is the main function of osteoclasts?

    a.   To break down bone tissue

    b.   To form new bone tissue

    c.   To maintain bone matrix

    d.   To regulate calcium levels in the blood

17. Where are osteoclasts located?

    a.   In the bone matrix

    b.   In the lacunae

    c.   On the bone surfaces in resorption pits

    d.   In the canaliculi

18. What is the lineage of osteoclasts?

    a.   Osteoblasts

    b.   Osteocytes

    c.   Monocytes

    d.   Lymphocytes

19. What is the function of prostaglandins produced by osteoblasts?

    a.   To break down bone tissue

    b.   To form new bone tissue

    c.   To maintain bone matrix

    d.   To regulate calcium levels in the blood

20. What type of cells are all bone lining cells?

    a.   Osteoblasts

    b.   Osteocytes

    c.   Osteoclasts

    d.   Monocytes

21. What are the two main parts of the female reproductive system?

    a.   Ovaries and uterus

    b.   Vagina and cervix

    c.   Fallopian tubes and uterus

    d.   Ovaries and vagina

22. Where does fertilization of the egg occur?

    a.   Ovaries

    b.   Uterus

    c.   Fallopian tubes

    d.   Vagina

23. What happens to the egg after fertilization?

    a.   It is implanted in the ovaries

    b.   It is implanted in the uterus walls

    c.   It is expelled from the body

    d.   It remains in the fallopian tubes

24. What is the purpose of menstruation?

   a. To release an egg from the ovaries

   b. To prepare the uterus for pregnancy

   c. To expel the lining of the uterus if pregnancy does not occur

   d. To regulate hormone levels in the body

25. What is menopause?

   a. The stage in which the reproductive system begins to produce female sex hormones

   b. The stage in which the reproductive system stops producing female sex hormones

   c. The stage in which the uterus is removed

   d. The stage in which the ovaries are removed

26. What is the function of the labia majora?

   a. To produce mucus secretion

   b. To enclose and protect other external organs

   c. To surround the openings to the vagina and urethra

   d. To allow sperm to enter the body

27. What is the function of the labia minora?

   a. To produce mucus secretion

   b. To enclose and protect other external organs

   c. To surround the openings to the vagina and urethra

   d. To allow sperm to enter the body

28. Where are Bartholin's glands located?

    a. Inside the ovaries

    b. Beside the opening of the vagina

    c. Inside the uterus

    d. Inside the fallopian tubes

29. What is the function of Bartholin's glands?

    a. To produce mucus secretion

    b. To enclose and protect other external organs

    c. To surround the openings to the vagina and urethra

    d. To allow sperm to enter the body

30. What is the purpose of the external structures of the female reproductive system?

    a. To produce eggs

    b. To allow fertilization to occur

    c. To protect genital organs from infectious organisms

    d. To regulate hormone levels in the body

31. What is bacterial vaginosis?

    a. A viral infection of the vagina

    b. A condition where the normal balance of bacteria in the vagina is disrupted

    c. A fungal infection of the vagina

    d. A condition where the uterus is infected

32. What is the most common vaginal infection in women of childbearing age?

   a. Chlamydia

   b. Gonorrhea

   c. Bacterial vaginosis

   d. Syphilis

33. What is chlamydia?

   a. A viral infection of the reproductive organs

   b. A bacterial infection of the reproductive organs

   c. A fungal infection of the reproductive organs

   d. A parasitic infection of the reproductive organs

34. How is chlamydia transmitted?

   a. Through the air

   b. Through contact with infected blood

   c. During oral, vaginal, or anal sex

   d. Through sharing of personal items

35. What are some symptoms of chlamydia in women?

   a. Painful urination and discharge from the penis

   b. Abnormal vaginal discharge and burning sensations while urinating

   c. Swollen testicles and fever

   d. None of the above

36. What are some symptoms of chlamydia in men?

    a.   Painful urination and discharge from the penis

    b.   Abnormal vaginal discharge and burning sensations while urinating

    c.   Swollen testicles and fever

    d.   None of the above

37. What is gonorrhea?

    a.   A viral infection of the reproductive organs

    b.   A bacterial infection of the reproductive organs

    c.   A fungal infection of the reproductive organs

    d.   A parasitic infection of the reproductive organs

38. How is gonorrhea transmitted?

    a.   Through the air

    b.   Through contact with infected blood

    c.   During oral, vaginal, or anal sex

    d.   Through sharing of personal items

39. What are some symptoms of gonorrhea in women?

    a.   Painful urination and discharge from the penis

    b.   Abnormal vaginal discharge and bleeding between menstrual cycles

    c.   Swollen testicles and fever

    d.   None of the above

40. What are some symptoms of gonorrhea in men?

    a.   Painful urination and discharge from the penis

    b.   Abnormal vaginal discharge and bleeding between menstrual cycles

    c.   Swollen testicles and fever

    d.   None of the above

41. What is the alimentary canal?

    a.   A passage through which food travels

    b.   A digestive chemical produced in the liver

    c.   An opening at the end of the digestive system

    d.   A small sac located on the cecum

42. What is the function of the anus?

    a.   To produce bile for digestion

    b.   To excrete waste (feces) from the body

    c.   To store partially digested food

    d.   To absorb nutrients from food

43. What is the appendix?

    a.   A small sac located on the cecum

    b.   The first part of the small intestine

    c.   The last part of the large intestine

    d.   A digestive chemical produced in the liver

44. What is chyme?

    a. A digestive chemical produced in the liver

    b. Partially digested food in the stomach mixed with stomach acids

    c. The first part of the small intestine

    d. The last part of the large intestine

45. What is the duodenum?

    a. The first part of the large intestine

    b. The last part of the small intestine

    c. A digestive chemical produced in the liver

    d. The first part of the small intestine

46. What triggers the salivary glands to produce saliva in the mouth?

    a. Chewing and breaking down food

    b. Smell of food

    c. Reflex action

    d. Voluntary control

47. What is the function of the esophagus?

    a. Mixing and grinding food

    b. Producing saliva

    c. Carrying food from the mouth to the stomach

    d. Absorbing nutrients from food

48. Where does swallowing take place?

    a. Mouth

    b. Stomach

    c. Pharynx (throat)

    d. Small intestine

49. What is the function of the stomach?

    a. Absorbing nutrients from food

    b. Breaking down food using enzymes

    c. Mixing and grinding food

    d. Producing saliva

50. What does the stomach secrete to continue the process of breaking down food?

    a. Saliva

    b. Bile

    c. Enzymes

    d. Acids and enzymes

51. What are the three parts of the small intestine?

    a. Duodenum, jejunum, and ileum

    b. Pharynx, esophagus, and stomach

    c. Cecum, ascending colon, and descending colon

    d. Liver, gallbladder, and pancreas

52. What breaks down food in the small intestine?

    a. Saliva

    b. Bile

    c. Enzymes released by the pancreas

    d. Acids and enzymes

53. Where are nutrients absorbed from food?

    a. Mouth

    b. Stomach

    c. Pharynx (throat)

    d. Small intestine

54. What is the function of the pancreas in the digestive process?

    a. Mixing and grinding food

    b. Producing saliva

    c. Breaking down food using enzymes

    d. Absorbing nutrients from food

55. What is the role of bile in the small intestine?

    a. Mixing and grinding food

    b. Producing saliva

    c. Breaking down food using enzymes

    d. Emulsifying fats for better digestion

56. Which group of vitamins includes vitamins B and C?

    a. Water-soluble vitamins

    b. Fat-soluble vitamins

    c. Minerals

    d. Folic acid

57. Which vitamin is essential for growth, healthy skin, and healthy hair?

    a. Vitamin A

    b. Vitamin B

    c. Vitamin C

    d. Vitamin D

58. Which vitamin is important for cell repair, digestion, energy, and the immune system?

    a. Vitamin A

    b. Vitamin B

    c. Vitamin C

    d. Vitamin D

59. Which vitamin is important for healthy body tissue, growth, cell repair, and immune system efficiency?

    a. Vitamin A

    b. Vitamin B

    c. Vitamin C

    d. Vitamin D

60. Which vitamin is important for healthy teeth and bones?

   a. Vitamin A

   b. Vitamin B

   c. Vitamin C

   d. Vitamin D

61. Which organs are responsible for filtering out excess fluid and substances from the bloodstream?

   a. Liver and gallbladder

   b. Lungs and trachea

   c. Kidneys and bladder

   d. Stomach and intestines

62. What is the function of urine in the urinary system?

   a. To filter out excess vitamins and minerals

   b. To remove excess blood cells

   c. To collect excess fluid from the bloodstream

   d. To aid in digestion

63. Which organ produces urine?

   a. Bladder

   b. Ureters

   c. Kidneys

   d. Urethra

64. Where are the kidneys located in the body?

    a.   Chest cavity

    b.   Abdominal cavity

    c.   Pelvic cavity

    d.   Cranial cavity

65. What is the shape and size of the kidneys?

    a.   Round and small

    b.   Triangular and large

    c.   Bean-shaped and about 4-5 inches in size

    d.   Oval and about 10-12 inches in size

66. What is the main function of nephrons in the kidneys?

    a.   Production of red blood cells

    b.   Regulation of blood pressure and volume

    c.   Digestion of food

    d.   Storage of urine

67. How are nephrons regulated by the endocrine system?

    a.   Through the release of hormones such as aldosterone, antidiuretic hormone, and parathyroid hormone

    b.   Through the release of enzymes

    c.   Through the release of neurotransmitters

    e.   Through the release of antibodies

68. What is the function of the renal corpuscle in a nephron?

    a.   Reabsorption of water and electrolytes

    b.   Secretion of waste products

    c.   Filtration of large solutes from the blood

    d.   Regulation of blood pH

69. Where is the glomerulus located in a nephron?

    a.   Renal tubule

    b.   Bowman's capsule

    c.   Vasa recta

    d.   Efferent arteriole

70. What happens to the excess blood that is not filtered into the glomerulus?

    a.   It passes into the efferent arteriole

    b.   It is stored in the bladder

    c.   It is reabsorbed by the renal tubule

    d.   It is transported to the liver

71. What is the role of the kidneys in maintaining water-salt balance?

    a.   Regulating blood pressure and volume

    b.   Producing red blood cells

    c.   Digesting food

    d.   Storing urine

72. Which hormone is responsible for the direct control of water excretion in the kidneys?

    a. Insulin

    b. Thyroid hormone

    c. Anti-diuretic hormone (ADH)

    d. Estrogen

73. What does ADH do in the kidneys?

    a. Causes insertion of water channels into the membranes of the cells lining the collecting ducts

    b. Increases salt excretion

    c. Decreases blood pressure

    d. Inhibits water reabsorption

74. What stimulates the secretion of ADH?

    a. Dehydration

    b. Ingesting water

    c. High blood pressure

    d. Low blood volume

75. Besides water, what else do the kidneys regulate in terms of salt balance?

    a. Excretion and reabsorption of certain ions

    b. Production of hormones

    c. Digestion of salt

    d. Storage of salt

76. What are kidney stones made of?

    a.   Bacteria

    b.   Red blood cells

    c.   Mineral salts and other waste products in urine

    d.   Hormones

77. What causes the formation of kidney stones?

    a.   Dissolved substances in the urine

    b.   Lack of minerals in the diet

    c.   Excessive fluid intake

    d.   Genetic factors

78. Which of the following is NOT a type of kidney stone?

    a.   Calcium stones

    b.   Uric acid stones

    c.   Struvite stones

    d.   Hemoglobin stones

79. What are some risk factors for developing kidney stones?

    a.   High fluid intake and regular physical activity

    b.   Family history of kidney stones and limited physical activity

    c.   Low fluid intake and a sedentary lifestyle

    d.   Young age and a vegetarian diet

80. What is a common symptom of kidney stones?

    a.   Blurred vision

    b.   Joint pain

    c.   Sudden pain

    d.   Loss of appetite

81. What is urinary retention?

    a.   Accidental leakage of urine

    b.   Inability to empty the bladder properly

    c.   Bladder infection

    d.   Weakening of the bladder wall

82. Which type of urinary retention requires immediate medical treatment?

    a.   Acute urinary retention

    b.   Chronic urinary retention

    c.   Urinary incontinence

    d.   Cystitis

83. What is urinary incontinence?

    a.   Inability to empty the bladder properly

    b.   Accidental leakage of urine

    c.   Bladder infection

    d.   Weakening of the bladder wall

84. What is cystitis?

    a.   Inability to empty the bladder properly

    b.   Accidental leakage of urine

    c.   Bladder infection

    d.   Weakening of the bladder wall

85. What is another term for fallen bladder?

    a.   Urinary retention

    b.   Urinary incontinence

    c.   Cystitis

    d.   Cystocele

86. Which medical field focuses on the study of hypersensitivity and allergies?

    a.   Allergology

    b.   Andrology

    c.   Anesthesiology

    d.   Angiology

87. Which medical specialty deals with male health and urological problems?

    a.   Allergology

    b.   Andrology

    c.   Anesthesiology

    d.   Angiology

88. What does anesthesiology primarily focus on?

    a.   Allergies and hypersensitivity

    b.   Male reproductive system

    c.   Induced state of amnesia and loss of responsiveness

    d.   Circulatory system and lymphatic vessels

89. Which medical field studies the vessels of the circulatory system and their diseases?

    a.   Allergology

    b.   Andrology

    c.   Angiology

    d.   Aviation medicine

90. What does cardiology primarily focus on?

    a.   Disorders of the heart

    b.   Oral diseases and their impact on the body

    c.   Male reproductive system

    d.   Induced state of amnesia and loss of responsiveness

91. Which medical field focuses on the diagnosis and treatment of diseases of the skin?

    a.   Dermatology

    b.   Endocrinology

    c.   Gastroenterology

    d.   Geriatrics

92. What does endocrinology primarily focus on?

    a.   Skin and its diseases

    b.   Diagnosis and treatment of endocrine organs

    c.   Diseases of the gastrointestinal tract

    d.   Health care of older adults

93. Which medical field specializes in the treatment and diagnosis of diseases of the gastrointestinal tract?

    a.   Dermatology

    b.   Endocrinology

    c.   Gastroenterology

    d.   Geriatrics

94. What does geriatrics primarily focus on?

    a.   Diseases of the nervous system

    b.   Diagnosis and treatment of cancer

    c.   Health care of older adults

    d.   Physiology, anatomy, and diseases of the eye

95. Which medical field specializes in the treatment and diagnosis of conditions and diseases related to the female reproductive system?

    a.   Gynaecology

    b.   Internal medicine

    c.   Microscopy

    d.   Neurology

96. Which medical field specializes in the diagnosis and treatment of disorders related to the ear, nose, throat, head, and neck?

    a.   Otolaryngology

    b.   Pathology

    c.   Pediatrics

    d.   Podiatry

97. What does pathology primarily focus on?

    a.   Disorders of the respiratory system

    b.   Medical care of children, infants, and adolescents

    c.   Study and diagnosis of disease

    d.   Treatment of arthritis and vasculitis syndromes

98. Which medical field specializes in the medical care of children, infants, and adolescents?

    a.   Otolaryngology

    b.   Pathology

    c.   Pediatrics

    d.   Podiatry

99. What does podiatry primarily focus on?

    a.   Disorders of the urinary tract and male reproductive system

    b.   Study and treatment of disorders regarding the feet and ankles

    c.   Scientific study of blood serum and other body fluids

    d.   Study of chemicals on living organisms

100.Which medical field focuses on the study of chemicals on living organisms, such as humans?

    a.   Psychology

    b.   Pulmonology

    c.   Toxicology

    d.   Urology

PART-THIRTEEN

ANSWER TO MEDICAL-ASSISTANT QUESTIONS

1. Answer: C

   Inorganic salts

2. Answer: C

   To support other organs and anchor muscles

3. Answer: B

   Flat bone

4. Answer: C

   Steel and iron

5. Answer: D

   Sesamoid bone

6. Answer: B

   To anchor muscles to bones

7. Answer: A

   Compact bone is harder than spongy bone

8. Answer: C

   Irregular bone

9. Answer: D

   To connect bones to other bones

10. Answer: B

    Flat bone

11. Answer: B

   To form new bone tissue

12. Answer: A

   Type 1 collagen

13. Answer: B

   To form new bone tissue

14. Answer: C

   To maintain bone matrix

15. Answer: B

   Lacunae

16. Answer: A

   To break down bone tissue

17. Answer: C

   On the bone surfaces in resorption pits

18. Answer: C

   Monocytes

19. Answer: D

   To regulate calcium levels in the blood

20. Answer: A

   Osteoblasts

21. Answer: A

   Ovaries and uterus

22. Answer: C

   Fallopian tubes

23. Answer: B

It is implanted in the uterus walls

24. Answer: C

To expel the lining of the uterus if pregnancy does not occur

25. Answer: B

The stage in which the reproductive system stops producing female sex hormones

26. Answer: B

To enclose and protect other external organs

27. Answer: C

To surround the openings to the vagina and urethra

28. Answer: B

Beside the opening of the vagina

29. Answer: A

To produce mucus secretion

30. Answer: C

To protect genital organs from infectious organisms

31. Answer: B

A condition where the normal balance of bacteria in the vagina is disrupted

32. Answer: C

Bacterial vaginosis

33. Answer: B

A bacterial infection of the reproductive organs

34. Answer: C

   During oral, vaginal, or anal sex

35. Answer: B

   Abnormal vaginal discharge and burning sensations while urinating

36. Answer: A

   Painful urination and discharge from the penis

37. Answer: B

   A bacterial infection of the reproductive organs

38. Answer: C

   During oral, vaginal, or anal sex

39. Answer: B

   Abnormal vaginal discharge and bleeding between menstrual cycles

40. Answer: A

   Painful urination and discharge from the penis

41. Answer: A

   A passage through which food travels

42. Answer: B

   To excrete waste (feces) from the body

43. Answer: A

   A small sac located on the cecum

44. Answer: B

   Partially digested food in the stomach mixed with stomach acids

45. Answer: D

   The first part of the small intestine

46. Answer: B

Smell of food

47. Answer: C

Carrying food from the mouth to the stomach

48. Answer: C

Pharynx (throat)

49. Answer: C

Mixing and grinding food

50. Answer: D

Acids and enzymes

51. Answer: A

Duodenum, jejunum, and ileum

52. Answer: C

Enzymes released by the pancreas

53. Answer: D

Small intestine

54. Answer: C

Breaking down food using enzymes

55. Answer: D

Emulsifying fats for better digestion

56. Answer: A

Water-soluble vitamins

57. Answer: A

   Vitamin A

58. Answer: B

   Vitamin B

59. Answer: C

   Vitamin C

60. Answer: D

   Vitamin D

61. Answer: C

   Kidneys and bladder

62. Answer: C

   To collect excess fluid from the bloodstream

63. Answer: C

   Kidneys

64. Answer: B

   Abdominal cavity

65. Answer: C

   Bean-shaped and about 4-5 inches in size

66. Answer: B

   Regulation of blood pressure and volume

67. Answer: A

   Through the release of hormones such as aldosterone, antidiuretic hormone, and parathyroid hormone

68. Answer: C

    Filtration of large solutes from the blood

69. Answer: B

    Bowman's capsule

70. Answer: A

    It passes into the efferent arteriole

71. Answer: A

    Regulating blood pressure and volume

72. Answer: C

    Anti-diuretic hormone (ADH)

73. Answer: A

    Causes insertion of water channels into the membranes of the cells lining the collecting

    ducts

74. Answer: A

    Dehydration

75. Answer: A

    Excretion and reabsorption of certain ions

76. Answer: C

    Mineral salts and other waste products in urine

77. Answer: A

    Dissolved substances in the urine

78. Answer: D

    Hemoglobin stones

79. Answer: C

   Low fluid intake and a sedentary lifestyle

80. Answer: C

   Sudden pain

81. Answer: B

   Inability to empty the bladder properly

82. Answer: A

   Acute urinary retention

83. Answer: B

   Accidental leakage of urine

84. Answer: C

   Bladder infection

85. Answer: D

   Cystocele

86. Answer: A

   Allergology

87. Answer: B

   Andrology

88. Answer: C

   Induced state of amnesia and loss of responsiveness

89. Answer: C

   Angiology

90. Answer: A

Disorders of the heart

91. Answer: A

Dermatology

92. Answer: B

Diagnosis and treatment of endocrine organs

93. Answer: C

Gastroenterology

94. Answer: C

Health care of older adults

95. Answer: A

Gynaecology

96. Answer: A

Otolaryngology

97. Answer: C

Study and diagnosis of disease

98. Answer: C

Pediatrics

99. Answer: B

Study and treatment of disorders regarding the feet and ankles

100. Answer: C

Toxicology

www.ingramcontent.com/pod-product-compliance
Lightning Source LLC
Chambersburg PA
CBHW082128290526
45794CB00008B/2967